THE ACCELERATED HEALING OF CHRONIC ILLNESS
Including Lyme Disease and Cancer

MAGENTA HEALING SYSTEMS –
An Evolutionary Approach to Taking Control of your Health

A GUIDE TO ACTIVATING YOUR INNER POWER

PEAK Results Coaching

Cover, Book & E-book Design by Velin@Perseus-Design.com

ISBN-13: 978-1-5346119-2-4
ISBN-10: 1534611924

Legal Disclaimer
The information contained in this book is the opinion of the author and is based on the author's personal experience and observations. The author does not assume liability whatsoever for the use of or inability to use any or all information contained in this book, and accepts no responsibility for any loss or damages of any kind that may be incurred by the reader as a result of actions arising from the use of information in this book. Use this information at your own risk. The author reserves the right to make any changes he or she deems necessary to future versions of the publication to ensure its accuracy.

This book is dedicated with Love and Gratitude for Deidy and Samuel

And to all those who are suffering in ways that we do not know and cannot understand.

CONTENTS

Warning...1
Welcome!...3
Why I wrote this for you...5

Magenta Healing System #1
Optimize the Foundation 9
    1. Tell Yourself the Truth 9
    2. Know What You Want 23
    3. Have a Plan to Get There 27
    4. Clear out the Clutter 31
    5. Take Control of Your Thought Life.................39

Magenta Healing System #2
Accessing the Healing State 43
    6. Love and Accept Yourself Fully 43
    7. Elevate Your Self Care.................................51
    8. Thought Dominance....................................69

Magenta Healing System #3
Water 75
    9. Self-Healing Strategies.................................75

Magenta Healing System #4
Imaging and Unfolding...83
    10. The Dynamic Process Unfolds.....................83
    11. The Dynamics Process Expands 97

Magenta Healing System #5 103
    12. Space and Fields 103
    13. 50 Rules for Healthy Living.........................113
    14. Summary..117

WARNING

The information provided in this report is for informational purposes only. It is the sole opinion of the author Jeff Forte, who has no formal health care training, holds no health licenses, nor health certifications.

This information is simply the opinion of the author based on his personal experiences. It is not intended to diagnose, treat, prevent, or cure any illness.

Never use this information as a substitute for the advice and guidance from a physician or licensed health care professional.

Always consult with a physician or licensed health care professional before starting any diet, exercise, or health care program.

How one person responds to any particular health related product or program might be different than the way others respond.

This information is never a substitute for any medication, treatment, or guidance prescribed by a physician or licensed health care professional.

WELCOME!

My intention with this book is to share with you what I have learned in recovering my personal health from a serious, chronic health challenge. You will read about that shortly.

Other insights have come from my work with others, including being a sole caretaker of 6 years for a family member with advanced cancer who is vastly improved and on the way to full recovery.

While none of these experiences were easy, they have given me a level of understanding about how to take control of your health that is unique, and potentially highly beneficial to you.

We have so many false assumptions, so many limiting beliefs, so much conditioning about what is and isn't possible. Yet miraculous recoveries occur. Unexplainable spontaneous remissions happen. People defy their diagnosis.

Not every cancer patient recovers from chemo, radiation and surgery, nor the variety of stem cell therapies, or Burzynski anti-neoplastins, or Gerson juicing protocol and raw food diet, or the countless other alternative procedures and processes available. Not every Lyme disease patient recovers with long term intravenous antibiotics, nor Advanced Cell Training, or any of the myriad of anti-microbial healing protocols out there, either traditional or alternative.

In my opinion, our understanding of each person's unique circumstances must evolve in order to help facilitate true long term health and vitality.

My goal is to give you immediately useful information that you can **use along with whatever healing protocol you have chosen.** These ideas have helped to amplify and accelerate my own healing, and other serious illness; including cancer.

Wishing you all the best in health,

Jeff Forte
PEAK Results Coaching

WHY I WROTE THIS FOR YOU...

At the peak of physical fitness in my life, I woke up one morning and knew something was very wrong with me. My legs felt strange and moving them was difficult. My brain was filled with fog. It was impossible to think straight.

When I tried to get out of bed, the room spun. I could not walk without holding onto the walls or I would fall down.

It's fair to say that I was scared. It would get much worse for me.

Was it a stroke? Was it Multiple Sclerosis, as some neurologists would believe?

Over the next eight years, I would lose my mind, my memory and my health, while chasing an actual diagnosis from some of the top medical experts all over the US.

My symptoms included monstrous migraine headaches, vertigo, exhaustion, inability to sleep, neurological tremors, impaired functioning in various organs and limbs, loss of high level brain functioning, memory loss, irregular heart beat and palpitations, body pain that would come and go, and constant dizziness.

There were a number of times I thought I was going to die. An emergency room physician confirmed my fears in one particularly bad episode with my heart.

When I had a few days of feeling a little better, and would run errands in my town that I had lived in for 18 years, I could not figure out how to get back home. All the memory of it was lost, and so was I.

It was emotionally devastating.

The simplest little things, I could not remember. My brain was shrouded in fog and there were times when I was literally unable to think. At other times my thoughts would be dark, ugly and completely uncontrollable. It was a nightmare beyond anything I could ever have imagined.

For eight years some of the best neurologists, infectious disease, and neuro-toxin experts in the medical community could not figure out what was wrong with me. It was frustrating, maddening, overwhelming, isolating, and depressing all at the same time. My health would improve from time to time and then the harsh setbacks would come.

Eventually, I would find out that I had struggled with severe, undiagnosed Lyme disease and dozens of associated co-infections for eight long years.

I want you to know about my past health nightmare, because I was able to completely overcome it. If I could do that, you too can begin to take control of your own health and ultimately your own healing.

While I don't have any idea of the specific struggles that you might be facing in your life, I do know this about you:

- **You are stronger than you realize.**
- **You are far more resilient than you might believe.**
- **And you are greater than anything you could ever face in your life.**

I want you to know that whatever health challenge you are going through; you have the ability to fully heal and more your life beyond wherever you are.

This is not a message of hope.

This is a message of absolute certainty that you can do this.

I want you to KNOW,…to absolutely KNOW with certainty, that you have untapped resources inside of you that can help you to accelerate the healing of chronic illness. These same resources are also available to help you to overcome whatever other challenges might show up in your life.

I'll tell you about some of those resources shortly.

By the way if you are curious, here's a list of some of the people I saw and the things that I did, over the course of a decade to get answers to my health crisis. Most of which did nothing for me. I did however collect an arsenal of information and experience.

It gives me a unique perspective and understanding of the variety of healing options, and modalities available. I did gather insightful wisdom along the way through my interactions with all of the following experts:

Cardiologists, Internists, Infectious Disease Specialists, Neurologists, Neuro-toxin Physicians, Integrative Medicine MD's, Lyme MD's, Naturopathic Doctors, Homeopathic MD's, Osteopathic Physicians, Chiropractors, and Energy Medicine Practicioners.

In addition, I have personally tried; Frequency Devices, Rife Machines, Onda Med, Hado Device, BioPhoton Devices, Advanced Cell Training (ACT), Biomats, Tesla Coils, Pulsed Electro Magnetic Field, Hyperbaric Chambers, Zappers, Acupuncture, Ozone, Infrared Sauna, Tui Na, Reiki, Pranic Healing, Tibetan Healing, Physical Therapy, Integrative Manual Therapy, Cranial Sacral Therapy, Lymphatic Drainage, Chinese Herbal Medicine, Traditional Herbal Medicine, and had countless blood tests and scans.

Unfortunately, I also had to learn about the world of healing cancer as the result of a family member's diagnosis. A similar multi-year journey was made to the top experts and clinics both inside and outside of the US. More wisdom was gathered about the traditional and alternative options available.

Both Lyme and cancer in my opinion have complexities that go far beyond the illness. Both traditional methods as well as alternative approaches of healing often fall short. This is simply true, or *everyone* from a particular protocol would be permanently healed.

That doesn't exist….yet!

Our understanding is evolving and the evolution of healing is just beginning.

A life is not healed by surgery, even though the surgery might be successful.

The primary focus of living must be to restore harmony in these four areas:

- Physical Health- We need balance in our bodies and in what we take into them.

- Emotional Health- We need to predominate peace, love and gratitude in our minds.

- Social Health- Our relationships play a sizable role in our personal wellness.

- Spiritual Health- We need to evolve ourselves, living lives of purpose and meaning.

Magenta Healing System #1
Optimize the Foundation

1

TELL YOURSELF THE TRUTH

The little things are the big things.

Let's take an honest look at your life.

You've got to have a starting point to begin your healing journey. No matter how bad things might seem, everyone has a beginning to their own healing. It can start today as you begin to implement some of the ideas that you are about to read.

Are you happy?

The United States might be the unhappiest country in the world. We fill over 260 million prescriptions for anti-depressants each year.

How happy are you on a scale of 1-10? (10 meaning you are filled with joy, and 1 meaning you're pretty darned miserable.)

Rate your overall life happiness and satisfaction. _____

As you might guess, unhappiness is a physical drain on health and vitality.

Happiness that comes from light playful moments or good things happening, is not enough for most people to feel happy with their lives overall.

In my opinion, it's also not enough to heal a serious illness.

Let's move beyond happiness;

What are you doing to find purpose and meaning in your life? These are the things that bring fulfillment, and an elevated state closer to joy, which begins to approach a healing emotional state.

What if we were here to develop ourselves fully, and to grow and evolve into the person that we are meant to be? Not just for ourselves, but to contribute to those around us?

Is personal growth and development important in your life? How would you rate your own progress and evolution to be a greater version of you?

How much stress are you under?

You already know that stress takes a very personal toll on us. What are you doing to deal with the stress of everyday life, not to mention the stress that comes from illness?

Do you have any rituals or routines in place to handle your daily stress?

If so, how effective are they?

Do they work well enough so that you can feel peaceful and replenished, with revitalized energy, at the end of your inner-calm inducing ritual?

It's important to understand that everyone needs counterbalances to the impact that emotional stress has on our health and vitality. We all need tools to help us cope with, and to offset the pace of our busy, hectic, pressure-filled lives.

How much time do you take to do something for yourself each week?

Your self-care has to become a priority if you want to accelerate your own healing. The excuses and stories of how you don't have time, and the rationalizations about why you aren't doing what needs to be done, only hurt you.

How physically fit are you?

Does it even matter?

According to the US National Institute of Health;

68.8% of adults are obese or overweight. 74% of men and 64% of women in the US are considered to be overweight or obese. And according to the National Health Institute, the associated health risks include: type 2 diabetes, heart disease, high blood pressure, nonalcoholic fatty liver disease (excess fat and inflammation in the liver of people who drink little or no alcohol), osteoarthritis (a health problem causing pain, swelling, and stiffness in one or more joints), some types of cancer: breast, colon, endometrial (related to the uterine lining), and kidney, and stroke.

You don't have to join a yoga studio, or lift weights or run marathons. Most any consistent moderate form of body movement is helpful to supporting your long term good health. Little things like walking, dancing, gardening, rebounding, and casual cycling are all beneficial. Simply find a way, any way to move your body more.

What rituals and habits do you have in place to move your body?

What does your daily food intake look like?

There is no question that what we eat and drink has a significant impact on our health and wellness. Decades of research indicate that reasonable daily dietary intakes of fruits and vegetables are beneficial to our health.

Directly from the US Centers for Disease Control (CDC)

Eating more fruits and vegetables adds nutrients to diets, reduces the risk for heart disease, stroke, and some cancers, and helps manage body weight when consumed in place of more energy-dense foods (1). Adults who engage in <30 minutes of moderate physical activity daily should consume 1.5–2.0 cup equivalents of fruit and 2–3 cups of vegetables daily.* However, during 2007–2010, half of the total U.S. population consumed <1 cup of fruit and <1.5 cups of vegetables daily; 76% did not meet fruit intake recommendations, and 87% did not meet vegetable intake recommendations.

How many servings of fruits and vegetables per day are you eating currently? _____

Is there room for more fruit and vegetables in your diet?

The evidence says that if you care about your health the answer is YES.

What do you drink?

Much like food, there are so many choices to consider: water, milk, soda, coffee, tea, alcohol, wine, beer, sports drinks, energy drinks, fruit juices, vegetables juices and combinations, etc.

According to the Harvard University School of Public Health, at least 50% of your liquid intake should be water. What percentage of your liquid intake is water?

Once you have decided to add more water to your diet, you still have choices. Do you choose tap water that might contain a variety of chemicals including fluoride, or bottled water that might have BPA and other chemicals in the plastic, or spring water, well water, reverse osmosis, distilled water, alkaline water or structured water?

Do you know the advantages and disadvantages in choosing one over another?

There is plenty of evidence that chronic dehydration is a factor in many health issues. Will you make drinking more fresh water part or your daily routine?

What's your job satisfaction like? (rated on scale 1-10, 10= love my job, 1=unhappy with current job,) _____

According to Forbes magazine and the Conference Board (a non-profit research organization) 52.3 % of Americans are unhappy with their jobs. That's an amazingly high number of people who are dissatisfied with their careers.

Is it healthy to do work that you don't enjoy, or work that creates personal unhappiness?

Of course not!

This also adds to the stress load that impacts your health.

You might be thinking, *"Hey Jeff I hate my job, but I can't find another one, so just what am I supposed to do?"*. This is why rituals around self-care and stress reduction matter. They play such a large part in allowing you to take control or your emotional well-being. Maybe you can't change your job, but you can begin to take control of your emotional health.

You'll learn about that later on in this book.

The ability to manage your emotional state will play an ever increasing role in your health as you age, because the impact of low level stress accumulates over time.

Are you happily married or in a satisfying intimate relationship?

Decades of research indicates that happy marriages result in increased longevity and lowered rates of serious illness. According to a study from Harvard Medical of 300,000+ people, they found that a lack of solid relationships increased the risk of pre-mature death by 50%; the equivalent of smoking 15 cigarettes per day.

You might want to read that again.

Relationship stress is not only unhealthy, it spills over into every other aspect of life, creating downward pressure on your energy levels and sense of well-being.

As an expert in relationship dynamics and the author of a book on marriage, *The 90-Minute Marriage Miracle*, I can assure you that many marriage challenges can be resolved reasonably quickly, even if traditional couples counseling has failed. If your marriage is struggling, the book will give you immediately useful ideas that you can begin to implement right away.

What are you willing to do about an unhappy relationship? Are you willing to consider the possibility that YOU need to do something more than you currently are. If your relationship isn't where you want it to be, realize this; any change starts with you.

Based on Harvard's study, for some people, that might turn out to be a life or early death type of decision.

What are your spiritual/religious beliefs?

I recently had a conversation with a man who didn't believe in God, nor hold any Spiritual beliefs about a higher power. This is perfectly fine, because believing or not believing in anything is simply a personal choice. Slightly over 3% of the US population is atheist.

When I asked him what did believe in, absolutely nothing came to his mind. In fact he expressed genuine concern when he couldn't come up with any answer at all, even after a few minutes of total silence. Interestingly, he had been meeting with me about the unhappiness in his life.

Did his lack of belief in anything greater than himself play a role in his unhappiness?

I certainly think so.

We all need something to believe in because it gives us a sense of perspective about the purpose of being alive. It can also give us a sense of belonging, like we fit into the bigger picture of our existence. When we believe in something greater than ourselves, it can add meaning to our lives.

Living a life that lacks meaning and purpose is certain to lack fulfillment.

There is plenty of scientific research that you can Google about quantum physics and the connection that we all share. There is also scientific evidence about the healing nature of prayer, as well as the health benefits of meditation. There is no question that any of these can be helpful at reducing and offsetting stress.

You could choose to believe in science, you could choose to believe in spirituality, or you could choose any particular religious belief, but you need to believe in something beyond yourself.

Do you have any rituals that provide you with a sense of peace or meaning, based on scientific, spiritual or religious beliefs?

Rate your level of overall life satisfaction? (1-10, 10 =loving my life, 1= empty) _____

Life satisfaction would include things like; your job satisfaction and success, intimate relationship happiness, physical health, emotional health, social connections, spiritual/religious/science based beliefs, and self-actualization.

To what degree are you living a life of your own choosing?

Do you feel empowered or disempowered, based on your current direction in life?

What would have to happen in order for you to feel that your life was more satisfying and fulfilling?

Are you willing to begin to pursue those things?

Maybe you are beginning to wonder, *"What does any of this have to do with healing any illness, including Lyme or cancer?"* From my perspective and personal experience, these are the pieces of the puzzle that help to facilitate true long-term healing.

Is your past conditioning and programming stronger than your desire to heal? Is your previous, possibly limited understanding of health, more important than learning and growing?

Years ago, a co-worker friend of mine was diagnosed with a brain tumor and had gone through surgery, and chemo-therapy. He was 35 years old, married with two young children, I was 24. He sat beside me and turned to me one day and said, *"It sucks when you know you're going to die."* I had no idea what to say.

That memory and the memories of numerous family members and close friends, who battled cancer and lost, are all permanently etched into my mind.

It also created plenty of motivation to search for some of the missing ingredient in healing.

We all know people who have suffered with horrific illness, and there is no shortage to the personal stories of family tragedies. I want you to understand that my experience indicates that other possibilities exist. There are things that you can do right away that are beneficial and elevating to your capacity to heal.

This book is for you.

Who do you rely on for emotional support?

Perhaps more than ever before, people frequently feel isolated and alone. While you might have 4,713+ Facebook friends and thousands of Instagram and Twitter followers, you could still feel completely alone.

Social media connections cannot fill the void of missing out on close personal friendships. We all need people that we can interact with in person who actually care about us, and that we genuinely care about as well.

Many people are hooked on their Facebook pages to see the updates of virtual friends as well as total strangers. People can spend countless hours scouring their news feeds and updates to distract themselves from the emptiness in their lives. To what end?

Who can you count on to be there for you in good times and bad. And who do you care about that you will be a true friend to, in fun times as well as the difficult moments that come.

All of the societies that are renowned for longevity; Abkazians, Hunzas, Okinowans, Ikarians, and Sardinians to name a few, make socialization with close friends an integral aspect of living a rich, healthy life. This isn't simply a coincidence. It's proof that living a long and healthy life includes having close personal friendships.

Is there room in your life for deeper friendships, and more genuine sharing of yourself with the people close to you?

Would it benefit you to expand your close circle of friends?

Rate your Physical and Emotional Health (Use that 1-10 scale for each, with a 1=Struggling and a 10= Excellent for physical and/or emotional health) Physical _____ Emotional _____

We all struggle from time to time physically and emotionally. As you already know, life throws challenges at us unexpectedly, some incredibly severe. And life won't stop giving us adversity that can shake us to our very core.

How we respond to the hardships and challenges of life, helps to shape who we become as individuals. Who you are today is a direct result of the meaning that you attached to all of your life experiences; both good ones and bad.

Some people use struggles to grow personally, and they find the inner resolve to overcome them. While others allow life's challenges to keep them stuck. The difference is simply the meaning that was attached to the challenges.

For example:

If you are struggling with an illness, what does it mean to you?

Does it mean that you might die, or does it mean that you have a chance at a fresh start to truly live your life? Which outlook would you prefer? Does it mean that you are depressed, or does it mean that you are committed to figuring out the answers, no matter how long it takes to recover?

Could you create a more empowering meaning to whatever challenge you might be facing in your life?

The impact of medications;

How many medications are you taking, and what are they helping you with?

Often multiple medications are needed to balance the side-effects of the original medication. Unfortunately you might also need one for the side-effect of the side-effect reducing medication. It can get crazy with even more medications to counter act the side-effects of multiple drug interactions.

According to the CDC over 37,000 people each year die from prescription drugs in the US. That's more than the deaths from illegal drugs or traffic accidents.

According to the Leapfrog Group, a national non-profit, and the US premier advocate for hospital transparency, up to 440,000 people die each year in the US because of preventable medical errors. That's an incredibly high number. In fact, I had to triple check it on their website. It's like losing a major city each year because of preventable mistakes.

While prescription drugs are clearly helpful to resolve any incredibly large number of conditions, ultimately it's in your best interest to work with your health care professional towards reasonable lifestyle changes that might allow you to reduce your dependency on the quantity and potency of your medications. *NEVER make adjustments to your prescriptions medications on your own.*

I repeat; NEVER make any adjustments to your prescriptions meds on your own.

Medications and emotions;

To what degree do you feel like you are in control of your emotional life?

Are you on any medications for your mental or emotional well-being? According to Medco Health Solutions, 1 in 5 Americans are now on at least one prescription drug for a psychological disorder.

These numbers drastically understate the real problem. People will also medicate themselves with pot, alcohol, or any other number of illegal drugs to numb or enhance their emotional states. There is no doubt that record numbers of people are pervasively unhappy and feel empty inside.

While medical marijuana can be helpful and is legal in a growing number of states, recreational pot use causes many problems. How do I know? Because I have young people in their early and mid 20's reaching out to me for help in resolving their pot habits. Many regular young pot users are coming to the realization that their unsuccessful, stuck lives are an empty mess.

Relying on a substance to escape your emotional life isn't healthy long-term.

I want you to know that no matter how bad things might seem, you have the potential to improve your situation dramatically. And in my opinion, a great deal of that will be up to you.

Your ability to control your emotional life has a great deal of influence on your health. Are you ready to learn how to take control of your emotional life? I will be sharing some specific ideas a little further on.

The honesty of where you are today is simply a starting point. It gives you something to build from. Hopefully it will also give you some perspective later on of just how far you have come.

Change can begin right now in this moment.

What changes would you like to make in your physical and/or emotional health?

Wanting something to change is not enough. Most people want to change some aspect of their lives, yet many are not willing to take the personal responsibility that creates change.

You must be willing to DO something different than you are doing today, in order for anything to change.

What are you willing to do differently in your life that might improve your health and begin to accelerate your own healing?

2

KNOW WHAT
YOU WANT

Lack of clarity gives us something else

I n conversations with clients I am often told what people don't want. It takes some real digging to get to what it is that they actually DO want.

Most often I hear that they don't want to feel stressed, they don't want to struggle, they don't want to be sick anymore, they don't want to feel sad, angry, frustrated, overwhelmed, unappreciated, unloved, disconnected, etc…

It's not enough to say, *"I don't want to have Lyme disease, or diabetes, or cancer, or MS, or osteoarthritis, or feel depressed, overwhelmed or angry."*

Knowing what you don't want is not a way to get what you DO want.

When you focus on what isn't working, and what is currently a problem, it keeps you stuck and unhappy. The only way out is to get absolutely clear on what you do want your life to be like, and begin to move towards it.

What exactly do you want your health to be like? What would your life look like every day, if you were vibrantly healthy?

Get clear about what you want your health and wellness levels to be.

- How do you want to feel every day?
- What do you want your energy levels to be like?
- What do you want your physical appearance to look like?
- What about the functioning of your mind and memory?
- How do you want to feel emotionally?
- What do you want your overall state of mind to be every day?

Clarity can be truly empowering. Do you have a compelling vision for your health and every other aspect of your life; including your relationships, your finances, your career, your social and spiritual life?

These are the big picture pieces of your life. And when you are focused on the big picture, the day to day typical life stressors tend to have less of an impact.

Realize this; it's impossible to have what you don't know you want.

Hopefully that previous sentence didn't melt any brain cells.

Take some time and actually write down the compelling vision that you want for your life. It could easily start with an inspiring vision of your physical and emotional health.

What does that look like for you?

Next; What's your WHY?

WHY you want something is just as important as knowing what you want.

Why do you want to be healthy and full of energy, what will it do for you? What will your life look like when you have restored or improved your health?

Is that an inspirational image?

You might be thinking, "He's getting carried away here, because doesn't everyone want to be healthy, and isn't that reason enough all by itself?"

Nope, it's absolutely not reason enough!

We all need something to look forward to. We need a reason to live. The suicide rates indicate that being alive is not enough reason to want to stay that way. Is it enough to want to live in order to go back to a horrendous marriage, or a stress filled and hated job, or an empty and lonely life?

We all need to have an outlook for the future that is brighter than our current life, because without that, where will the inspiration to change our situation come from?

If your life is a dead end what's the point of recovering your health, if only to go back to an unhappy life?

Find a reason to live. Discover something within you that says ENOUGH! That there is more than the life I am living and I will recover my health to move my life far beyond whatever exists today.

At one point in my Lyme illness, when it wasn't possible for me to walk even 50 feet without stopping, I decided that one day soon I was going to run on the beach with my son. At the time it was a fantasy, but I absolutely knew it would happen, and the idea of it was very inspiring to me. It was everything in the difficult moments.

It took 4 years, but I was finally able to run on the beach with my son. In that moment, the elation that I experienced, and the feeling of personal victory, was one of the most profound emotional feelings in my life.

I want you to have that same experience of elation when you create your very own personal victory.

Give yourself a truly inspiring vision of the future. Have something special in mind to motivate yourself and be willing to do whatever it takes to recover your health. Keep the reason you want to be well in your mind as often as possible. Focus on creating that brighter tomorrow simply one day at a time and one moment at a time whenever needed.

I saw this quote many years ago and it has stuck with me;

"While the difficult takes time, the impossible just takes a little longer".

My particular vision didn't have a time limit, I was willing to work on it every single day until it was fulfilled, and no matter how long that took.

Why do you want to recover your health? To do what exactly?

What's your WHY?

Create a new vision of your future in your mind. See yourself doing exciting things, and being healthy and happy. Imagine the feeling of completely recovering your health.

How important and meaningful is achieving this vision to you?

3

HAVE A PLAN
TO GET THERE

Having no plan might just be a plan to fail.

How is your health vision going to happen?

- What specifically are you going to do?

- How will you evaluate whether it's working or not?

- How will you stay on track and know if you 're making progress?

- What will you do if it's not working, or if significant setbacks happen?

- Who will you rely on for help and support?

Yes you definitely need a plan with specific strategies to help yourself heal. And you certainly need to work with health care practitioners that you trust and believe in, who also have a track record of success. I found some that were very helpful to me in understanding the priorities of what needed to be done.

In my personal situation, while I had made some progress with a variety of alternative health care providers, I was frustrated with the pace and rates of improvement. I didn't feel like I was getting the help and answers that I really needed. I had been struggling far too long, and it seemed like my money was going out much faster than I was improving.

My search looking for help outside of myself was over. I no longer had any desire to continue seeking answers from the medical community.

Yes, that's right; I stopped seeing all MD's and alternative health care providers. I made a decision to take complete, personal responsibility for my own healing.

***This is absolutely a bad idea for most people. I highly recommend you stay with a physician or licensed health care practitioners that you trust and believe in. There are lots of caring, highly competent people out there. Find one that can be a true partner in your healing. Your belief in your treatment plan as well as your physicians, are integral components in your healing success.

In my situation, even though I was helped by some of the professionals that I saw, I simply wasn't getting the full results that I wanted, and I was fed up with wasting my time and money. In addition, I had accumulated enough knowledge and understanding, over years of researching and talking to experts, to know just what I needed to do. I was totally confident in my ability to help myself heal. Not one doubt existed in my mind.

Soon after I started working on my own healing, my results began to accelerate, and my symptoms and condition began to improve. Eventually all of my symptoms and the Lyme disease itself would be gone. To confirm my beliefs, I was tested several times for traces of Lyme and none were found.

The big picture of my own healing plan included removing the underpinnings of the disease. That required an upgrade of my thinking and understanding. It also included; healing

body, mind and spirit; while making dietary changes, mindset shifts, offsetting hidden emotions, detox of parasites, metals and chemicals, immune system rebuilding, killing Lyme bugs and co-infections, healing and rebalancing organs and systems, and striking a delicate balance between Lyme microbe die-off and still being able to function, restoring inner alignment, and repairing energy centers and fields.

Clearly not everyone needs all of this in order to heal. Fortunately I did, so that today I have a much higher level of understanding about healing chronic illness.

In my opinion, staying healthy long-term requires permanent upgrades in your nutrition intake, your thoughts and feelings, your physical movement, your life balance, your environmental awareness, a connection to something greater than yourself, and an upgrade to social and family interactions.

You will read about some of the specific things that I did for myself a little further along.

- What are you going to include in your healing plan?
- What will be your daily priorities?
- Who will be your health recovery partners?
- What will be the most important components of your plan?
- Which aspects of your plan will you be personally responsible for?

4

CLEAR OUT THE CLUTTER

Is what you are doing helpful,
supportive and beneficial for your health?

Let's start by taking a look at your refrigerator and kitchen cabinets. What will we find to eat and drink in there? How many highly processed, high sugar and nutrient depleted foods will we find in your home?

My own vision is to achieve and sustain optimal health. If your vision or goal is to heal yourself from an illness or disease, it's essential that you evaluate the impact of what you are taking into your body for nourishment.

- ✓ **Do the foods you eat help you to prevent, heal or recover from illness?**
- ✓ **Do the liquids you drink support your body's immune system?**
- ✓ **Do you eat high quality nutrient rich food?**

Let's look at a real life example:

Does a McDonalds Big Mac with a large order of fries, and Coca Cola support my health goal? Does it improve my body's ability to heal? Is it beneficial to my health? In my opinion, definitely not.

Does eating a cream cheese bagel, snacking on candy and potato chips, and drinking high sugar energy drinks while adding a hamburger, sausage and peperoni pizza, support my body's ability to heal? Is that helpful to me? Again, I don't think so.

Lots of typical American food choices add inflammation to the body, which delays healing, and contributes to a variety of diseases.

Here's what I did:

I figured out which diet would work for me by testing a number of them. You could do the same thing. For example; I have been gluten-free for over 12 years. Why?, because I feel better than when I was eating gluten.

Over the past 12 years I sampled for months at a time; being a strict vegetarian, a vegan, and a raw vegan. However, I didn't like how I felt with those diets. While I did feel lighter, I also felt weaker. My body seems to do better with small amounts of selected proteins; herring, organic turkey or grass fed buffalo.

I don't eat red meat, pork, chicken or eggs. Why?, Because I feel better if I don't. I also don't eat fish other than a few wild caught Haddock or Cod a few times a year. Why? Because so many types of fish contain high levels of contaminants that I prefer not to take into my body.

I made all of my dietary choices primarily on only two things;

1. **What felt right for my body by testing it out or intuitively knowing.**
2. **Based on the research that I've done about the best healing foods.**

I also chose more vegetables; drank fruit and vegetable smoothies, drank only clean, structured well water or spring water. I ate lots of beans and lentils, and as I mentioned some lean proteins with more vegetables. I would occasionally have quinoa, or sprouted, gluten-free, multi-grain bread with a meal.

I eliminated all processed food, all sugar, and any food with even a trace of sugar in it, all high carbohydrate foods; like breads, pastas, white rice and white potatoes. I reduced my meat protein intake and avoided all processed meats.

Why?

Because in my opinion those types of foods did not support my body's ability to heal. And that is exactly what I wanted and needed. I wanted to be as supportive to myself as possible, so I chose to monitor my dietary choices from a new perspective.

This was an incredibly easy decision for me.

My health mattered so much more to me than any past habitual food item that I might have enjoyed. And to all you bacon lovers out there, Yes, I even gave up bacon.

I ate and drank only what in my opinion would sustain my body's ability to heal.

By focusing only on nutrient dense foods, in as close to their natural state as possible, I was able to give myself the nutrition that my body needed to help it recover.

Let's keep things simple for you.

Does your current intake of food and drink; support or benefit your health and life force? Are you taking in only what's helpful and beneficial to your body?

Are your food choices helping to clear your health issues out, or are they clogging you up and keeping the illness stuck?

Clearing out your thought clutter.

Certain emotions are elevating to your mood while others are detrimental. Certain feelings support your health, while others diminish it.

Positive emotions like: love, peace, joy, happiness, bliss, elation, laughter and gratitude are elevating and healing.

Negative emotions like: despair, loneliness, emptiness, hopelessness, depression, rage, guilt, shame and resentment are depleting and suck energy from your body.

- What are the predominant feelings of your thought-filled day?
- Are you aware of the primary thoughts and feelings that you habitually hang out with?

Do they uplift you, or bring you down?

Our lives are driven mostly on auto-pilot based on our past emotional programming. Very few people have any idea of how many negative thoughts and feelings that they have on any given day.

We must begin to become conscious of the thoughts that we have, and make an ongoing effort to reach for a better feeling, moment by moment. As we become more aware of what we are experiencing our emotional lives can begin to improve.

For example:

- Anger is a better feeling than depression, because anger in the short term creates a desire for action. Anger could become a catalyst to defy a diagnosis. Depression tends to keep us stuck. It gives us no movement forward at all.
- Peace, on the other hand is a more elevated emotion than anger because it brings inner harmony. In the moment you feel peaceful,

any and all stress has vanished, and that's a very good thing for your health.

- Love is also a much more elevated and empowering healing emotion than either anger or sadness. The feelings of love are beneficial to the chemical processes in your body.
- Laughter can also be beneficial. Author Norman Cousins in his book Anatomy of an Illness talks about how he used laughter to help himself heal from a terminal illness.

Is it possible to love, laugh, or inner peace yourself back to health?

I personally know that it is. Both love and peace were components in my own healing.

If it was possible for me, and it was possible for Norman Cousins, and countless others; isn't it possible for you too?

If you are caught up in a negative cycle of thoughts, simply begin to change your focus by remembering something funny, or peaceful, or sensual, or blissful, or loving. You could replay in your mind the feelings of a past personal victory. Continually reach for a better feeling and you will break the cycle of negativity in short order.

This does require your conscious choice.

You have to decide that you will monitor your thoughts and feelings more closely. Be on alert to catch the negative thoughts that show up, and then consciously choose an elevated thought that feels better.

If you do this consistently as part of a new daily routine, soon your thoughts will begin to become more and more positive all by themselves. Your mind will begin to reorient itself towards better thought feelings.

Clearly there are no side effects in doing this other than you will feel better emotionally, and potentially begin to feel better physically. So why not start today?

Clean up Your Stressors

We all have things in our lives that increase our stress levels.

- Are there certain people that habitually irritate you?
- Are there interactions with family members that create feelings of anger, frustration, anxiety or guilt?
- Are your finances a mess and creating bad feelings inside of you?
- Do you hate your job?
- Do you feel stressed-out simply thinking about work or co-workers?

In order to bring balance back into your life, these are the types of things that need to be offset or eliminated.

What habits and rituals could you adopt that would create more inner harmony in your life?

- What makes you feel good?
- What makes you feel at peace?
- What types of things could you do for yourself that makes you feel re-energized?

Create a daily routine for yourself that allows you to feel good more often. You could start with the smallest thing as long as it improves your emotional experience;

You might stare into a flower for 3 minutes. You might feel the sun on your face. You might smell cinnamon for 10 seconds. You might walk in nature, or on the beach, in your backyard, at a park, along a stream, etc… You might call someone you care about and tell them you love them, without talking about anything else other than how much you care about them. You might visit a place that has butterflies. You might stand barefoot in the grass and look at the clouds or look at the stars. You might close your eyes and focus on your breathing... in ...and out as you consciously relax every part of your body starting with your toes and working your way up.

You are only limited by your willingness to be creative.

What small things will you do for yourself starting today?

In addition to exercise, I meditate almost every day for 15-20minutes. Because I have been doing this for several years, any stress that I might experience during the day or previous day is immediately let go.

Find something that brings you inner peace, and be willing to test out any number of ideas to determine for yourself what works best.

You could also try yoga, tai chi, getting a massage, reflexology, any form of meditation, guided imagery, painting, jig saw puzzles, gardening, ca-ressing a pet, shared times with loved ones etc...This should all become part of your healing plan, and there is much more ahead.

5

TAKE CONTROL OF
YOUR THOUGHT LIFE

*Your thoughts can either propel your forward or hold you back.
They can create a life of happiness, or daily suffering.*

I f you do a Google search on the impact of emotions and health, you will find plenty of scientific research that suggests negative emotions contribute to health challenges. The opposite is also true; positive emotions have a positive influence on our health and well- being.

I won't bore you with all the research, but big things like heart disease and little things like healing blisters, are all impacted by our emotional state. The more you examine the research, the more you understand that choosing to experience positive emotions will lead to better health outcomes.

Let's look at those little blisters for a moment.

Ohio State University found that in an induced tiny blister experiment; having a 30 minute argument with your spouse can delay your healing by a day. If you argue regularly, the healing time doubles. When couples talked about areas of disagreement, the healing time took up to 40% longer.

You can sense that this begins to have important and potentially life-altering implications. This is also more proof that your personal

health can be influenced by the happiness level of your intimate relationship.

Maybe this is a wake-up call to the reality that our subtle emotional lives have an enormous impact of our immune systems, and overall health and vitality. Do some research on the subject for yourself and it will truly open your eyes, perhaps motivating you to finally take control of your own emotional fitness.

- **Is long-term chronic stress beneficial to your health?**
- **Is being unhappy all the time supportive to your immune system?**
- **Is feeling guilt, anger and shame regularly, useful in recovering from illness?**

The answer is NO, so please do yourself a favor and work on cleaning up your emotional clutter.

Our bodies are easily capable of handling small amounts of stress. And clearly we are able to handle significant stressors once in a while.

It's the non-stop stress that many people experience over long periods of time that slowly erodes their immune system, and adds degenerative chemicals like cortisol into the blood stream.

If instead we begin to feel the feelings of gratitude, peace and love, these emotions would add different chemicals like the anti-aging, hormone precursor DHEA, into the blood stream.

Which chemicals are you choosing for yourself with your emotions; ones that might be healing and anti-aging, or others that might be degenerative and health eroding?

With this basic understanding, the conscious choice becomes easier.

I had a moment of clarity that helped me to finally take control of my own healing from chronic Lyme disease.

I began to consider the possibility that if I simply loved myself fully, completely and unconditionally, that my Lyme disease might go away.

We will get into some of the things that I did about that shortly.

- **Are your thoughts creating empowering or disempowering emotions?**
- **Are your thought elevating to your life experience?**
- **Are your daily thoughts helpful, and beneficial to your healing?**

What from this section will you add to your personal healing plan?

6

LOVE AND ACCEPT YOURSELF FULLY

How you feel about yourself is what matters the most.

This inspiring theme became a foundational force in my personal healing solution. And I believe that it can potentially help you as well. Certainly there are no down-side risks, and no debilitating side-effects if you add this idea into your own healing plan.

A note of caution; even though this might look and seem simple enough, it isn't necessarily easy for everyone. At times some people have found it challenging.

Why might it be difficult to love and accept yourself fully?

Everything that has happened to us in our lives; all of those experiences and all of that information, has been stored and recorded in our unconscious minds. It's there in the background constantly driving and limiting our lives.

Imagine that you carry an enormous white board around with you every day.

On this white board is written everything that you have ever heard about yourself, and any thought that you've had about yourself. Maybe it's 48 years' worth of written thoughts. There's probably lots of stuff on that white board that isn't particularly empowering or supportive to you. Unfortunately you are consciously unaware of almost all of it, but it is impacting you whether you want to believe it or not.

As part of my own healing, I needed to erase lots of those old thoughts off of my white board. In addition to making peace with and offsetting many emotions that I was unaware of, elevating my level of self-love was essential to shifting the balance of white board thoughts into my healing favor.

Most of us have plenty of old evidence that says we aren't worthy of loving and accepting ourselves either fully, completely, or unconditionally.

This might be why:

Maybe no matter what you did, it was judged as not good enough, or maybe you were rejected by someone you truly cared about and it diminished how you feel about yourself, or maybe someone said something bad about you, and that has stuck with you and limits you even today.

Maybe at some point in your life you weren't smart enough, or talented enough, or attractive enough, or fit enough, or successful enough, or rich enough, or perfect enough, etc...

Do you constantly compare yourself to others?

Did some injustice happen in your life that still has a hold on you today?

There are plenty of reasons why someone might find it difficult to love and accept themselves at the level that might initiate or accelerate healing.

Do you secretly desire that someone else will love and accept you uncon-ditionally, so that you will finally be able to feel good enough about you?

If so, you will forever be disappointed.

Often I speak with people who have taken their own self-worth and un-knowingly given it away to someone else. Not realizing that they can only feel worthy and deserving of love if that other person loves and accepts them *enough*. It can become a desperate longing to be loved and valued by anyone else but you. It's an impossible task.

Imagine that. Someone else gets to decide that you are worthy of love. Imagine that you have based your entire value as a human being on some-one else's opinion.

That is a recipe for a life of unhappiness.

If you have ever done this, right NOW is the time to begin to take your power back.

Decide… that from this moment on, no one will ever take an ounce of your self-worth away from you. No one will ever again get to decide that you are worthy of love. No one will ever be able to have you believe that you aren't good enough for the things that you want in your life. And no one, absolute-ly no one but you, will ever determine your value as a person.

Today, you can begin to take ownership of your self-worth, and that starts with loving yourself a little bit more.

Understand that it is SELF worth, SELF love, SELF esteem, SELF confidence, and SELF value.

Only YOU get to decide any of this, and not any other person on this earth.

You are absolutely worthy of love, and deserving of the life you choose to pursue. You have gifts and abilities that make you unique and special. You are a precious gift to the world.

I honor all of that in you. And I want you to begin to honor that in yourself.

It starts right here, right now, with a new decision that comes with complete inner resolve. It's that feeling of inner strength that says, ENOUGH! You have that inside of you and so much more.

Here is how you can begin to love and value yourself at higher levels.

This brief 7 step exercise helped me to accelerate my own healing:

This simple exercise can be done in just 3-5 minutes a day.

Of course it can be done for any longer amount of time, but I want to eliminate your excuse of; *"I don't have the time."*

Anyone can find 3-5 minutes. Right?

1. **Find someplace quiet and comfortable to sit or lie down.** Anyplace quiet will work as long as you won't be interrupted. There is no right or wrong about how to do this exercise. There is only doing it so that it feels good for you.

2. **Close your eyes and begin to scan your body.** In your mind simply take a look around from a place of curiosity. What do you see and feel? What are you aware of? What sensations do you notice?

You could begin at your feet and work your way up towards your head, or start anyplace you like. Simply scan your body and see what you feel, and become aware of any sensation that stands out.

Do you feel pressure, discomfort, tingling, numbness, blankness, etc, in any particular areas of the body? Whatever you feel, just notice it, and nothing more.

Do this now. Close your eyes for 25 seconds and scan your body and see what you become aware of.

You will scan your body again for a second time after this exercise, and simply notice any changes that might have occurred.

That's it. Scan your body, notice what you notice, and scan it again after the exercise below and see if anything has changed. That's all there is to it.

By the way, any change is good. Anything not changing is also good. Whatever you are aware of is good. There is no other judgment or evaluation needed. Just be curious and let go of anything else.

After you have scanned your body...

3. **Tell your body and numerous parts of your body that you love it.** Simply say *"I love you my body"* and actually feel love and gratitude for your body for 7 or 8 seconds. You could say it out loud or silently. Be thankful for your body serving you 24 hours a day, all year long. Sometimes we forget all the work it does for us.

Now, you will tell as many body parts as you want that you love them too, in any order of your choosing, pausing 7- 8 seconds for each part... again, no right or wrong of any choice.

For example say or think: *"I love you my brain"*, and feel love and gratitude for your brain for 7-8 seconds....then, *"I love you my heart"*, and feel love and gratitude for your heart for 7-8 seconds.

And continue *"I love you liver"*, and feel love and gratitude for your liver. *"I love you lungs."* and feel love and gratitude for your lungs. *"I love you thyroid*", and feel love and gratitude for your thyroid, *"I love you my immune system*", and feel love and gratitude for your immune system.

And continue with any organ, system, or gland that you choose, one at a time.

Continuing Example: "I love you stomach, chest, back ,spine, nervous system, eyes, spleen, face, skin, legs, gall bladder, arms, hands, kidneys, ears, thymus, knees, pituitary, ankles, etc.....

It is the FEELING of love and gratitude that you want to feel for that body part. It's not about mumbling the words to get through the exercise. Take an intentional 7 or 8 seconds for each part and FEEL love. If you can't feel love, you can certainly FEEL grateful for that part for being there for you and working so hard for you. Continue with the exercise.

There is no perfect order, or right or wrong order, no right or wrong body part. Any order or body part that you choose to love is perfect.

You could easily get all the major organs and body parts done in 3-5 minutes. You might find that you notice certain feelings when you love a particular organ. You might not. Anything that you notice or feel is welcome and perfectly Ok.

4. **Scan your body again when you are finished with loving the body parts.** Scan it in the same way that you did in the beginning. Just look around from a place of curiosity for any new sensations or subtle shifts or changes.

5. **Have awareness-** What did you notice? Did anything change? Do you feel any different? Did you notice anything at all that stands out differently now? How did it feel to do this exercise?

6. **Make this a new ritual in your life.** Do this at about the same time every day or multiple times a day. Again no right or wrong. Do what feels best for you. I did this mostly once a day, on occasion twice/day.

7. **You must bring the FEELINGS of love and gratitude into this brief meditation to the best of your ability, or you are wasting your time.** Take the full 7-8 seconds or longer to direct those feelings at each body part.

I want to reiterate that you can scan your body in any order. You can love your body parts in any order you prefer. You can love different body parts or go into more detail on any given day. There is no right or wrong. Go based on what feels best at the time.

There were days when I would get into more details and find deeper layers to love and appreciate. However, every day I would connect with all of the major organs that I thought would influence my healing.

Try this for yourself daily for at least 30 days.

I am still doing this little exercise several years after healing myself from Lyme because I sincerely believe it has helped me as well as the people I have taught it to.

Please give this little act of kindness to yourself the chance you deserve.

Here's a brief summary:

1. Find someplace quiet.
2. Close your eyes and scan your body.
3. Tell your body and numerous parts of your body that you love it and are grateful for it. Go Slowly.
4. Scan your body again

5. Have awareness, what changed if anything? Be curious.
6. Make this a daily ritual
7. Make sure you bring the FEELINGS of love and gratitude into the exercise.

This is the beginning of being able to love and accept yourself at higher levels. There is more ahead. Pay attention to the subtleties of how you feel before, after and during this mini-meditation.

Set aside the time and actually go do this.

Do not underestimate the impact of this because it's only 3-5 minutes. Find out for yourself over the course of 30 days what the impact is on you.

7

ELEVATE YOUR
SELF CARE

Is what I'm doing depleting,
supporting or elevating my health and vitality?

A realization occurred to me early on in my self- healing adventure, after I had already made a bunch of changes. I had to consider the possibility that I wasn't actually doing enough to heal myself.

So I began to look at things in very simple yet transformational terms:

Is what I'm doing; Depleting, Supporting or Elevating my health and vitality?

This was then applied to every aspect of my life.

Let's get specific:

Will the food I normally eat; Deplete, Support or Elevate my health and vitality?

This was a reality check for me. I thought I was doing Ok, and I was. I also wasn't doing enough. There was another level needed.

My honest answer was that my normal diet, even though it was decent, was primarily at the supportive or beneficial level. While it wasn't diminishing, it was only occasionally elevating. I believed that in order to heal myself, I needed my food choices to be Elevating to my life force.

I made immediate changes to upgrade and optimize my nutrient intake, and settled into a diet that was about ~80% raw and organic foods, I upgraded the quality of my supplements to raw or natural state. I also chose a variety of sprouted foods, fermented foods, wild plants and superfoods, to further elevate my body's level of nourishment.

If people thought I was a health nut before, I just brought a whole new level of food fussiness into my life. And I continue to eat this way.

After all, didn't I deserve the best quality that I could find?

Don't you?

And yes, it was and is more expensive.

However, it was far less expensive than continuing to pay doctors and take their incredibly high priced supplements.

Simply do the best you can while upgrading your choices.

I juiced organic wheat grass frequently and juiced organic, fresh vegetables daily. My smoothies became even more nutrient rich with a variety of raw, green plant powders and select superfoods. I chose many supplements and foods based only on their nutrient density. I cut back further on my meat protein intake and ate more organic legumes. As a result of these elevating changes, I began to achieve an optimal level of nutrition for my body's healing.

As you may recall, I eliminated all sugar, fried foods and processed foods.

Eliminating these foods was easy for me because I equated eating sugar with feeding Lyme spirochetes, and I couldn't imagine doing that to myself. I haven't cheated once on that commitment to myself in over 8 years.

I can't imagine ever eating sugar, or any food item containing sugar, again in my life. I will not do it. This is just a personal choice.

You will also decide what is best for you.

If you are wondering; why be so extreme?

I eliminated sugar and the other foods because they are not Elevating to any aspect of my health and wellness.

In my opinion sugar can only be in the *Depleting* category, so to stay true to my commitment it must be avoided.

To be certain that I avoid sugar and other ingredients that might diminish my health, I became a food label fanatic. Sugar is everywhere in processed food choices, and so are any number of chemicals and artificial ingredients that you might want to avoid.

I also severely limited my eating out at restaurants.

You need to be aware that many restaurants use significant amounts of sugar in their meals. This was a huge surprise to me. The truth is that sugar use in restaurants combined with low cost, low quality ingredients, puts many of the food choices in the; *Depleting to your health category.*

Because the quality of the food nutrition at most restaurants was significantly less than I could provide for myself, it made little sense to eat out, other than a few particularly high quality primarily vegetarian choices.

Are you this committed to yourself?

To me, this isn't about right and wrong, or that this particular item is good and that one is bad. It's simply about eating; Health Diminishing, Health Supportive or Health Elevating foods. It's been a highly effective choice-point filter for me.

Simply decide what makes the most sense for you, and follow that path to the best of your ability.

We all have incredible inner resolve when we decide that something is worth it. You could close the door today on your favorite food item and never eat it again. But you must have a truly compelling reason why you would want to do that.

For me the choice was simple; did I want to regain my health, or stay sick?

I chose to elevate my health, and naturally my diet had to reflect that path immediately.

What food changes, if any, will you make in order to get to the Elevate category?

Is your reason for making any dietary changes compelling enough?

How will you benefit? What's in it for you if you change your diet?

Some people equate eating this thing or that, to a matter of life or death. It keeps them tenaciously committed. Others have decided that wanting to live to fulfill an inspiring purpose is reason enough to make the dietary changes they want. People have used scientific or research studies to validate their choices, or relied on local health experts.

I never looked at my dietary changes as; I HAVE to do this...

It was always; I WANT to eat this way and I'm Going to!

What matters is that your food choices work for you. There is no right or wrong about whatever you decide. Do what you feel is best for you based on whatever criteria you choose to rely on.

Give your choice a powerful meaning that inspires you to stay with it. Normally a balanced diet with moderation of a variety of food choices is perfectly fine. However when you are battling a serious illness, that is unlikely to be enough to accelerate your healing.

Dietary changes by themselves were definitely beneficial to me. I did feel better after elevating my food choices. They were just not enough for me to heal fully. I needed to do much more.

Elevate Your Thoughts

The thoughts we think have a direct impact on our immune systems, and the optimal functioning of our body's energy systems.

What does that actually mean for you?

You learned earlier on that scientific research has shown negative thoughts and feelings are depressive to our immune system. While on the other hand, positive thoughts and feelings have been shown to support health and longevity.

You might say that the happy optimist is indeed healthier, and lives longer on average than the unhappy pessimist.

Are you thoughts; Depleting, Supportive or Elevating to your mood?

Do they lift you up or make you feel bad?

Managing your emotional state when you are sick, or sick and tired of being sick, is not always an easy thing to do.

Any negative thoughts and feelings might have plenty of evidence to support them. However, remember that negative emotions are depleting to your immune system. They are depleting to other energy systems of the body, and create chemicals that are also gradually depleting to health and vitality.

If you are feeling overwhelmed, depressed, angry, hopeless, empty, frustrated, fearful or alone, the best thing to do is simply reach for a better feeling.

Can you think of something in your life that you are grateful for?

You could FEEL grateful or thankful for big things, little things, or anything at all.

For example:

You might FEEL grateful that the grass is soft, or that the sky is blue, or that you have electricity, or that you have water to drink, food to eat, a car, a tooth brush, sunshine, windows to look out, plates for your food, a phone, a TV, the color pink, a roof over your head, toilet paper, eyes to read this, etc....there is no end to things that you could feel grateful for.

Will you choose to find things to feel thankful for?

And remember, you have all of those parts of your body that you can feel grateful for as well.

Gratitude is an elevated emotion that you will find beneficial to your emotional wellness.

Another component in my healing plan was to go over a list of things that I felt grateful for before I went to sleep. Why? In order to create better healing chemicals for the night.

This took only 2 or 3 minutes. It was easy. It's also very easy not to do.

What about you, will you add the gratitude exercise before you go to sleep each night?

How will you remind yourself every day to do what you are learning in this book?

The Emotion of Love

Love is a highly elevated emotion that causes more healing chemicals to flow.

There are different aspects of love. You could feel love for a spouse, a child, a friend, a pet, the ocean, the stars, a plant, the connection that you have with God or the Universe, etc....

Slow down and take a moment to do the following;

Think of a time when you felt love.

Feel that feeling in your body as if you were there, in that exact moment when you felt love. Be there fully; imagining that moment once again... re-living the feeling of love.

Notice what you feel in your body. Notice the location of the feelings of love. Now magnify these feelings of love... breathe them in more fully and more deeply...Make the images you see in your mind brighter... make the images even larger. Feel the feelings of love expanding within you...immersing you...surrounding and bathing you in love.

Please take a moment to do this. It will give you an experience of how you can enhance healing feelings.

You did do this little exercise right?

If you took the 9 seconds to do it, now focus on the subtleties of the feeling changes in your body, before vs. after. I want you to understand that it doesn't take very long at all to shift our emotional state. However, it does take consciously choosing to make it happen.

There is healing power in the feeling of love, so call on it often to lift your emotional state.

My thought about; *loving myself fully, completely and unconditionally* became a healing tool, and a gateway to creative experimentation. There were noticeable levels of depth to the subtleties of the impact of loving my body parts and organs. I discovered that more and more was possible from what looked like a simple little exercise.

I realized it was far more than that.

Bringing love into my body became a highly complex getaway to a zone where resolution of previous challenges was possible. There was a stillness that occurred in the subtleties that seemed to allow larger and more rapid shifts to occur.

I also realized that at certain levels love could easily blur into the feeling of peace. And I did find deep levels of peace within the feelings of love that I also utilized for healing.

Feelings of Peace

Can you think of a moment when you felt truly peaceful?

Maybe you were in nature, or listening to beautiful music, or petting your cat, or getting a massage, or walking on the beach, or sitting in the sunshine, or taking a relaxing bath, or holding someone you love, or sitting in a rocking chair chewing 11 pieces of bubble gum while staring into a fire. (I did that many years ago, and it was incredibly peaceful for me at the time.)

Peaceful moments can come in unexpected ways. Peace is another powerful Elevated emotion that you will find beneficial to your mood, and helpful in producing chemicals that offset stress and other disempowering emotions.

Deep Inner Peace creates a stillness, where one internal reality has the potential to blur into another. In my experience, this can be used to offset past emotional traumas and more.

If you bring a curious mind into the layers of your own healing journey, you will discover that many fascinating possibilities exist within the experience. This allows you to access more and more of your own healing power. The more you do it, the easier and deeper it gets.

The Value of your Sense of Humor

Think of something funny.

Can you remember a moment when you just laughed out loud. Maybe someone did something or said something that had you rolling in laughter. Sometimes kids laugh so hard that milk comes out of their nose. Have you ever had the giggles, when you just couldn't stop laughing? Have you ever doubled over and laughed so hard that your stomach hurt?

Humor is a useful gift for healing. *As someone said, laughter might just be the best medicine.*

Find humor in life. Find humor in yourself.

We can make life way too serious, and it's easy for us to get caught up in our own pain. I've certainly been there wallowing around in my own self-pity. Doing that never offered any help, so I never stayed very long.

If you are feeling sorry for yourself, how is it serving you? How is it serving the people around you?

In the famous words of Abraham Lincoln; *Live, Laugh, Love, Learn and Lighten the F**K up*.

Ok, maybe Abe didn't actually say that. But I heard the expression many years ago and adopted the; *lighten up*, aspect for myself.

Could you benefit in any way by being more lighthearted?

Are you fun to be around? Do people enjoy your company even if you are struggling with an illness? Do you bring lightness or feelings of heaviness to the people around you?

Our minds give us the ability to change our focus in an instant. When we change our focus, we can also change our emotions.

For example:

Think about something that's bothering you…..Got something?….So think about that thing that bothers you.

Now think about something that you are proud of, or think about something that you worked really hard for and accomplished, that filled you with personal satisfaction.

If you are thinking about the feelings of pride or accomplishment, you are no longer thinking about that thing that bothered you. Your brain can only focus on one thing at a time, giving you the ability to shift your thoughts and mood upon your choosing, creating a more uplifting healing emotional state.

Reach for a better thought-feeling continuously throughout the day, and your overall mood will brighten for your own empowerment, and the fun of those around you.

Breathing

Most of us are not breathing optimally. If you watch a baby or young child breathe, you notice that only the belly is moving. Not the chest.

Having worked with clients who had panic or anxiety attacks, I can tell you that breathing rises up into the chest under stress. The more the stress, the higher in the chest, and the more shallow the breathing.

Do this:

Place your hand over your navel, and gently and normally begin to breathe into your navel, allowing your hand to help target your breathing. Do not force your breathing. Do not exaggerate your breathing. Utilize your normal soft, gentle and natural breathing, and simply allow it to go deeper into your lower stomach and navel area.

Do this for 30 seconds.

Now tune into how you feel. Do you feel any different? If you are feeling stressed out or overwhelmed, breathing normally into your navel area will help to reduce some of those feelings. You will feel slightly better. For some people, significantly better.

Try this out for yourself. Use this simple tool to help yourself to take a little more control over your emotional life. Do this lower stomach navel-breathing intentionally, many times throughout the day for just 30-90 seconds. If you do this enough times, you will retrain your breathing back into rhythm with what is more supportive to your health.

Rebounding

This is something that I do daily.

A rebounder is a round device that looks like a mini-trampoline. Some rebounders have a bar attached that you can hang onto for support, while others do not. Bouncing on a rebounder is called rebounding, and it's a great addition to your healing plan.

NASA research found this device to be the most beneficial of all exercises in helping astronauts restore bone mass when returning back from outer space. In addition, they found that gentle bouncing or rebounding was beneficial in the following ways:

- Boosts lymphatic drainage and immune function
- Great for skeletal system and increasing bone mass
- More than twice as effective as running without the extra stress on the ankles and knees
- Increases endurance on a cellular level by stimulating mitochondrial production (these are responsible for cell energy)
- Rebounding helps circulate oxygen throughout the body to increase energy.

Not all rebounders are created equal. The one you might buy at Walmart will not be as effective as one of the sturdier more expensive models. The one that I use has metal springs. I do not suggest a rebounder with bungee cords for suspension. Look for one with at least a 250+ pound weight limit.

Electro Magnetic Fields (EMF's)

You may realize that we are being bombarded with EMF's. Some people are more sensitive to things like cell phones, cell towers, computer screens, wireless devices, WI Fi, 3G,4G, cordless phones, satellite transmissions, and dirty electrical fields, etc…

There is evidence that EMF's can be depleting to health, particularly for sensitive individuals. Find out for yourself.

Here's what I do to avoid unnecessary EMF's after I realized that I had a sensitivity to them. I was easily fatigued sitting in front of my computer after a few hours. I didn't like the feeling I had when holding a cell phone to my head. I don't sleep as well if my Wi Fi is on.

- I changed all of my cordless phones to old fashioned wired phones.
- I don't use my cell phone for phone calls, or even keep it in my pocket for more than minutes unless it is turned off.
- I unplug the WiFi in my house at night.
- I will not use a computer without an earthing/grounding mat
- I sleep on an earthing sheet and often take it with me when I travel.
- I go barefoot often to get the benefits of the energy field of the earth.

In my own situation, reducing my exposure to EMF's has been elevating to my health.

Sunlight

In my opinion, sunlight has numerous healing and balancing properties beyond creating vitamin D in the body. Imagine what happens to life on earth without sunlight.

There is evidence that sunlight helps with sleep cycles, depression, strengthens the immune system and is preventative against a number of diseases. Obviously you want to avoid excess amounts of sunlight, because too much can be harmful. Find the balance that works best for you.

I get out in the sun without sunglasses as often as possible. Even in the middle of winter in the Northeast, I try to get out in the direct sun for 15+ minutes whenever possible. Sunlight definitely feels beneficial to my overall health. I do suggest avoiding the mid-day sun in summer and personally prefer to experience the rays of the hot summer sun during the morning or later afternoon.

Earthing

There is a great book to read on the benefits of earth energy. Much as we require sunlight to thrive, we also require a connectedness to the earth's energy field. With the advances of modern society, we are exposed to less and less earth energy. We are constantly disconnected from this vital energy field.

I highly recommend this book; *Earthing; The most important health discovery ever?*, *by* Clinton Ober, Dr. Stephen Sinatra, and Martin Zuker. A variety of Earthing products are available on Amazon and other places.

I no longer fatigue when sitting in front of my computer for hours at a time, because I use an earthing/grounding mat. The difference in how I feel efore using this mat and after, is truly remarkable. They only cost about $40, so it's well worth trying out for yourself.

Connecting to the earth helps to remove inflammation from the body. That's a very important point to ponder. A variety of elite athletes use earthing technologies to help their bodies recover faster from training and competitions.

Proper Breathing, Reducing EMF exposure, experiencing sunlight on your body and utilizing the grounding energy of the earth are all ways to help elevate your self-care. They are absolutely worth adding to your healing plan.

Muscle Testing

This concept has been incredibly helpful to me. It has saved me time, money, and allowed me to focus on what food and supplements are most beneficial for me.

The operating principle behind my muscle testing is that I only want to take into my body what is good for me, and to avoid things that are not.

This was a simple, yet incredibly profound light bulb idea for me. It has been truly transformational in my approach to healing and honing in my own intuition.

One of the side benefits of muscle testing, is that I have greatly enhanced my own inner wisdom about what is needed, both for myself and often with clients.

Please review this section carefully and visit youtube.com to see a demonstration.

The origins of muscle testing come from applied Kinesiology or Bio-Mechanics. It's the use of muscle strength to identify weakness and imbalances in the body. It can also be used to identify beneficial nutritional supplements to offset imbalances.

While the traditional medical community does not view this as scientifically beneficial, I personally encountered numerous traditional and alternative physicians using a variety of muscle testing techniques to evaluate me, and determine what supplements might benefit me.

It took me months of practice to finally be able to muscle test for myself. The reason it took so long is that I wanted to do it my way, not the way that would actually work. It never occurred to me that being right handed and wanting to do what was most comfortable, was the opposite of what would work. I thought I simply needed more practice.

I tell you this to open your mind to other possibilities in case one preferred way isn't working.

One day in frustration of not getting it, I decided to switch to my left hand dominant and I was able to muscle test instantly. I had wasted lots of time with my own silliness and closed minded focus on how I wanted things to be.

I hadn't been open to the possibility that it would work the opposite way. A highly valuable lesson was learned...the hard way as usual,...again.

Here's what I do;

I make two O rings with my thumb and middle fingers using low-medium strength, and interconnect the circles, linking them. My left linked ring is the solid foundational ring that always remains closed. The right linked ring may open or close as I gently pull the rings apart with a specific muscle test that I might be doing.

Please watch this on youtube.com using a search for *linked ring muscle testing* there. You will see a number of very short videos walking you step by step through how to do it. There are also numerous other methods that you can evaluate by searching *muscle testing* on youtube.

I am able to test supplements and foods as to whether something is good for me in that moment or not. My right hand O ring will go weak if something isn't good for me, and I will be able to sever the linked finger connection without doing anything consciously myself.

If something is good for me, the right ring will remain solid and I won't be able to pull them apart. This is like holding something on my body and asking "Is this good for me." I then get a yes or no answer based on the linked rings remaining solid or linking broken.

It's kind of like creating your own finger chain, asking a question, and then gently pulling the circle links apart, without changing the level of strength holding the finger circles together. If they hold; for me that means yes, if they separate; that means no.

Why do I use my middle finger with the thumb and not another finger? Because that's what works best for me, having tried out all the other fingers.

You have to be willing to experiment and find out for yourself what will work best for you. Youtube is the best place for short videos, with the step by step instructions of exactly how to do it.

Practical Application of muscle testing:

When I was more recently bitten by that tick, I knew that I would want to use some of my anti-microbials to kill the Lyme spirochetes and co-infections. I happen to have well over a dozen of them.

Which one is best at any given time? How much do I take? Which ones won't help me?

Muscle testing allowed me to know which specific anti-microbials would be best to use, and how many drops of each would be most beneficial for me. This process is highly dynamic. What worked well in the morning, might no longer test well for me later on that day. Another anti-microbial might be needed in a different amount.

To clean up the lyme bugs, I ended up using a total of eight different anti-microbials in varying amounts. I never used all eight on any given day. Typically, a unique set of 4-5 different antimicrobials were able to eliminate most of the spirochetes and co-infections.

Let's imagine for a moment that you think this is nonsense.

That's perfectly Ok. I willingly support your process and whatever works for you.

For me, the proof is obvious. I was able to heal myself quickly. And I feel great using the supplements that muscle test well for me. The people that use this method for a variety of illnesses are able to target for themselves what their bodies need at any one time.

Is it simply a *placebo effect*? Is it simply that I and others believe it works, so it does?

What you are reading comes from my own healing path of discovery. If any of this information doesn't resonate with you, be ok with that. Use what feels right for you and honor your own wisdom.

There is no one path for healing. There is no one size fits all when it comes to treating and permanently resolving chronic illness.

You are being given a menu of choices that you will decide for yourself what to take and what to leave behind.

Be open to anything that might be useful in your healing while honoring your own path.

You are going to visit youtube.com and take a good look at *muscle testing* for yourself aren't you?

8

THOUGHT DOMINANCE

A decision can be made that closes off every other possibility,
Allowing only the one you want to occur.

I n my opinion in order to heal yourself or accelerate your own healing, you must have one of the following in your dominant thoughts:

Love Peace Will

You have read about my thoughts on the healing benefits of laughter, love and peace. My personal healing journey began with the power of Will.

I knew that I was going to heal, and I was willing to do anything and everything possible to make that happen. I had an intense inner resolve about my full recovery. My mindset, or will to live, was strong. My will to survive my symptoms on any given day was high. I refused to allow myself to die, although there were a number of times that I truly worried it was actually going to happen.

In those moments, I would access an inner reservoir of determination and find more resolve. This internal refusal to give into my symptoms, no matter how severe they might be in any moment was not always easy. I did it anyway. So too can you.

There is this place inside of you, perhaps at the very inner core of your being, which allows you to handle whatever life throws your way. The will to survive, the will to continue on, the will to rid yourself of your unpleasant circumstances is within all of us.

There is a warrior within you willing to wage battle relentlessly for as long as it takes. Never complaining about how difficult the struggle might be; only resting from time to time in order to fight on with a renewed sense of tenacity and resolve. Honor that warrior part within you.

Can you Will yourself back to health? My own experience is proof that it is possible.

Ultimately, my healing was a combination of Will and Self-Love that often blurred into Peace. I also discovered that Laughter naturally increased in my life as I embraced love and peace more frequently. Those are all empowering, healing emotions, but my path started first with my will to survive, along with an unwavering determination to defy my illness.

Hope Believe Know

When you think about your illness or challenge, I believe that there are only 3 categories of possible thought dominance.

- **You could Hope to make a full recovery.**
- **You could Believe that you will make a full recovery.**
- **You could Know that you will make a full recovery.**

While hope is a more elevated emotion than despair or hopelessness, in my opinion it is not enough to create healing. Unfortunately, hope is also not a strategy for success.

To me, the feeling of hope lacks strength. It lacks resolve. There is very little to hold onto. It contains nothing solid and therefore cannot be the foundation of your healing plan.

I hope...I hope....I hope...

I want you to hope that the sun comes up tomorrow. Say to yourself, *I Hope that the sun will come up tomorrow.* Notice the feeling.

Now say to yourself, *I Believe that the sun will come up tomorrow.*

Does believing feel stronger than hoping? I think so. Thinking you are going to heal and believing you are going to heal are both more empowering than hope.

There is an even more empowering feeling than believing.

Now say to yourself, *I Know that the sun will come up tomorrow.*

Compare the; *I know the sun will rise tomorrow*, with the *I believe the sun will rise tomorrow*, or the *I hope the sun will rise tomorrow*, which one feels more certain to you?

I *knew* that I would heal. I never *hoped* to heal myself. That felt like weakness to me. I did believe and think it would happen, but I absolutely *knew* that it was truly possible for me to do it. Doubt did not exist in that *knowing.*

If it was possible for me or anyone else, it is certainly possible for you.

I want you to wrap yourself in a blanket of KNOWING that healing is truly possible for you. Why would it not be possible? Even if the so called experts say that the odds are low or even nil, it is STILL POSSIBLE.

People have miraculous healings, unexplained spontaneous remissions of all forms of illness that cannot be medically explained. It baffles the medical profession. Doctors do not have all the answers. They are not able to predict YOUR future.

The *placebo effect* is a well-known, scientifically documented phenomenon that allows healing to occur from something as simple as a sugar pill. Can you create your own personal placebo effect? Did I? Because almost anything is possible, your ability to completely recover is one of those possibilities.

Feel that *Knowing it's possible to heal*, deep into your heart and your stomach. Get your brain focused on Knowing that it is in fact possible. Feel the inner strength in knowing that your own healing is possible. Now use this knowing feeling every single day, and to the best of your ability, go do your part.

When you know, truly know, you have elevated your own capacity to heal. What then remains to be done are just the little every day details.

Self-Evaluation

What are the criteria that you will use to judge how you're doing?

I highly recommend that you judge yourself only on your EFFORT. Your effort to do your best about any of the following things:

Your EFFFORT to elevate your diet, your EFFORT to elevate your mindset, and your EFFORT to experience Peace, Love or Will, while KNOWING that your healing is possible every single day. Judge yourself on your EFFORT to fully do your part to heal.

And be willing to cut yourself some slack if you had a lousy day. No one is perfect particularly me, and I had many moments that were less than ideal. Vow to be better the next day and endeavor to deliver on that vow day after day.

Give yourself a daily grade if it helps. Was your diet an A+ effort today or a C-. Was your emotional state an A or a D because you wallowed in self-pity? Did you skip a day of self-love? If so, get yourself back on track now.

Can you look yourself in the mirror at the end of the day and say that you truly did your part to the best of your ability?

There is nothing more than that.

However as I discovered, what I actually could do, was beyond what I had been doing. When I realized this incredibly important point, I saw more and more opportunities to rise up out of my own limitations.

There are many outcomes in life that you cannot control, but you can control your daily effort to have whatever you want.

Right now in this moment, make a vow to yourself. Make a very personal, internal commitment, with all the resolve that you can muster. I'm wondering what that will be?

You have the potential to tap into, and honor, a greater aspect of yourself than you realize.

Magenta Healing System #3
Water

9

SELF-HEALING
STRATEGIES

Our willingness to explore the possibilities and
limits is only the beginning.

You are about to read some of the exact strategies that I used to help accelerate and resolve my chronic Lyme disease. These strategies have also been helpful to a large assortment of illness and disorders. If you have a healthy sense of skepticism that's perfectly ok, but it can also get in the way of your own healing.

Simply keep an open and curious mind about the following concepts and strategies. They have proven themselves to work for me and many others that I have taught them to.

Give them an *honest* try for yourself, go all in, and see what happens.

Anticipate Your Healing

Bring the feeling of anticipation into your life. Anticipate your healing with joy and gratitude. Know that it's arriving any day now, and that its' arrival is inevitable. Imagine the feeling as if you are already healed. Feel that gratitude in your body. Feel the joy. Anticipate doing the things you will be doing having fully recovered already.

I focused on the feeling of running on the beach with my son. I did this more often as a reminder to myself when I felt horrible. I saw it. I felt it. And I experienced it my mind every single day until it actually happened. I anticipated it happening and brought the feeling of actually doing it into my body frequently.

The Power of Water

A number of years ago I had a chance to see Japanese scientist Dr. Masaru Imoto talk about his book *Hidden Messages in Water*. It expanded my thinking. He showed how the influence of our thoughts, words and feelings on molecules of water, can positively impact our personal health.

Yes, our thoughts, words and feelings on molecules of water, can impact our health.

Let's imagine for a moment that you don't believe this to be true. Still skeptical?

Researchers all over the world have proven that water is able to carry memory and information. With a simple Google search you can verify this. And there is active and ongoing scientific research to explore the properties of water, and the potential capabilities that the molecules of water contain.

You might be thinking, *"Ok maybe it has been scientifically proven that water is able to carry memory and information, but what does that have to do with me?"*

The average human body is about 60% water.

What if that water is actually carrying memory and information inside of you?

And I began to wonder about the memory and information that my body's water might carry. Was it supportive to my health? Was it positive?

Did it even matter?

What about all of the negative thoughts that I had been having, what about all the thoughts I wasn't aware of, were they impacting my body's water, and ultimately influencing my health?

I had no answers for my own questions.

If our bodies are around 60% water, I realized that this water was circulating into every area of my body, bringing messages and information to cells, organs, systems and molecules.

This *light bulb* moment of realization was enough to get me to do something about it.

The curiosity that I have spoken about a number of times, was just the motivation needed to experiment with my body's water.

I began to talk to my water.

If you remember in the previous chapter *Love and Accept Yourself Fully* I talked to my body and my organs. Talking to my water was just a continuation of what I was already doing to a degree, but at an elevated level.

I started to tell my water, *"I love you."* Then things got interesting.

How would I know if it was working? I wanted some type of actual proof that it was working.

I had an idea, could I visualize a representation of my own inner water?

I asked my mind to show me an image of my body's water. A small lake appeared in my visual mind. It looked similar to a lake that I knew well in Vermont.

I noticed the image of the water, noticed the appearance of the water, and noticed the color and clarity of the water, and the scenery around the water.

I was just the curious observer...and then I said, *"I love you."*, and instantly ripples appeared in the water.

This was BIG!

While you might be thinking; *your mind just made that up, or maybe it didn't really happen.* To me it was my proof that my water was responding to my thoughts/words. Whether I was unconsciously changing my water in the image, or my water was changing in the image, or I imagined the entire thing, didn't matter to me.

I didn't care HOW or WHY the water changed. I only cared that it did.

Having studied the work of Dr. Milton Erickson, an American psychiatrist and psychologist, who specialized in medical hypnosis and transformational therapies, I had a hypothesis. He was famous for his paradigm setting work with the unconscious mind. I remembered reading that he trusted the unconscious minds of his patients 100%.

The ripple in the water could have been created by my unconscious mind responding to me, so I simply trusted it 100%.

The more I talked to my water image, the more it changed. There were times that I wasn't able to see the image. It seemed to disappear only to reappear a few days later. There were no patterns to what was happening, other than things were definitely changing in, and to the water. I was also feeling a little better overall.

What was making the difference in how I was feeling? I didn't care what it was, I only cared that I was feeling better. I attributed it to the accumulation of all the care taking that I was doing to my body, organs, and water. But something new was definitely working for me.

Here's how to do this simple process:

You are going to use similar steps to saying *I love you* to your body and organs.

1. **Find someplace quiet. Close your eyes.**

2. **Tell your mind to show you a visual image representation of your body's water.** It might be a stream, a river, a pond, a lake, an ocean…etc. It could be anything that isn't water. It might be a truck or a flower or absolutely anything at all. Be Ok with whatever image pops into your mind. Be Ok if no image pops into your mind. There is no right/wrong or good/bad.

3. **Direct the thought out loud or silently, *"I love you."* into the image of your water.** If you have no image, simply direct the thought intentionally into your body's water.

4. **Feel the love and gratitude for your water.** Tell your water how much you appreciate it and feel the love for your water. Do this even if you can't see the water. I have had people who did not get

an image originally, be able to see a visual impression of their water later on.

5. **Notice what happens; something changes or nothing changes, with the image of water.** Be Ok with either one. Simply be curious, nothing more.

6. **Tune into the feeling that you get from the water.** Is there an emotion seemingly attached to your water? In the silence and peacefulness can you tune into a feeling, or sense of intuition that your water needs anything from you? One day I had the feeling/intuition that there was anger in my water. So I simply told my water that I was sorry and that I only wanted peace for it. I said, *"I bring you peace."*, and felt peace for my water... and then immediately the small waves on the surface of the water disappeared and the color brightened.

7. **Be Patient and Focus on the Big Picture.** Simply bring the healing emotions of love, gratitude, forgiveness, or peace into your water. Be on the lookout for any subtle changes, because they will give you the sense that you are on the right track.

8. **Thank your mind for the image of your water even if you don't see it yet.** Thank your water again for being there for you. Once you have done that, you are done for the moment.

9. **Combine this with the body and organ conversation that you are already having.** Take an extra 90 seconds or more with your water in combination, or take several minutes communicating with your water all by itself. There is no right or wrong. Do what feels right intuitively for you.

This was only the beginning.

I found water to be a truly unique, dynamic access point for transformational change. In my experience, the changes that occur in the water, even small changes, seem to create changes in the physical body and/or mind.

Sometimes there is a lag time with no rhyme or reason, and at other times, the changes are reasonably fast and potentially almost immediate. While this is far from a perfect system, it has proven to be truly beneficial in my own healing as well as clients.

While I have extensive experience and understanding of my work with water, I recognize that what I know today will expand and evolve even further, as additional layers of application reveal themselves.

The more I worked with my water, which I still do even today, the more I realized that there was much more to be done with my body's organs, and systems to accelerate my healing.

The conversations with my water, body's organs and systems, would become much more involved, intricate and dynamic.

I had discovered another level of exciting potential to accelerate my healing from within.

Magenta Healing System #4
Imaging and Unfolding

10

THE DYNAMIC PROCESS UNFOLDS

*What we think we know pales in
comparison to what is unknown to us.*

As my water and I got more acquainted with each other, things began to show up in the water. Sometimes it was debris of some sort, at other times a film would be on the surface, or objects in the water. There were times the water was extremely cloudy and dirty looking, and once in a while, the surface of the water would become very rough with large waves.

On more than one occasion there were particularly unusual things in the water. I saw a variety of bugs and small critters that I couldn't identify. I didn't freak out. I simply accepted whatever appeared without offering any judgment on it.

I realized that this was only my unconscious mind creating things for me to address. So I trusted them 100% as something to work on.

My goal was always to make the water crystal clear and serene. Honor you own wisdom and intuition about how your water should look.

It was rare if that happened early on, but I was always able to improve the appearance. Sometimes the water would get stirred up, only to settle back into a peaceful appearance 10 seconds later.

For those who are able to imagine your water in your mind, how you see it in the beginning will change later on. How much later? It could be a day, a week, or 3 months. There is no way to know, because your unconscious world operates completely different than anyone else's.

For those who are not able to see their water in their imagination, that's Ok. I mentioned that I am not always able to see the image of my water, so I found some other markers.

One way to know if this is working for you and are unable to visualize an image of water, is to scan your body before and after the conversation. You may be aware of a slight feeling shift in your body, or even a profound change in a localized feeling in a particular part of your body.

Look for evidence from the subtleties of your feeling awareness, for proof that something is actually happening.

Do you feel any differently before and after talking with and loving your water?

Another reminder, as long as you are being positive, loving, kind, peaceful and offering forgiveness etc…this process will benefit you.

Imagine that you are talking to a very important part of yourself. Obviously you only want to say kind, loving, positive, empowering and beneficial things.

*Never say anything negative to any part of your body or water.

If, in the past you have done so from time to time, not to worry. It can all be cleaned up with loving, and peaceful thought conversations with your body and water. Unintentional mistakes are Ok, because they can be corrected.

The original image that I had of my water was a lake, and that lasted in different forms for a few months. Eventually the image in my mind turned into an expansive ocean. Why? I don't know, and again, I don't need to know. Certainly I have ideas about that, but because I simply trust what exists, I am always able to let go of having to figure out why this, or why that. That's an endless loop without anything beneficial resulting. So, avoid it.

I am completely accepting of whatever shows up in my minds impression of my water, including sea monsters, which actually did appear in my water one time. It was a non-event, only something to be addressed.

Clients working with me have expressed to me seeing images of people, images of weird objects, trucks, rocks, images of plants, birds, trees, toys, spiders, butterflies, etc…,and colors and textures of the water all across the visual spectrum.

If you see something bizarre, it is perfectly normal. If you see something you don't like, it is perfectly normal. Remember though, the idea is not to judge whatever is there, but to simply accept it as something to be resolved. If you see something that doesn't make sense, it is all perfectly normal and consistent with my experience.

I would not be surprised by anything you might tell me that showed up in your water. In fact, I would be eager to hear about any of the strange things that might have actually appeared for you in case it might help me figure out another facet of the system. Email me at jeff@peakresultscoaching.com if you get anything truly fascinating.

I accept whatever is there and work with it. I highly recommend you do exactly the same thing. Nothing more is ever necessary.

So far, everyone's water changes at a different pace in a different way. Based on my observations and the feedback from clients, there is absolutely no connection to what happens in any one person's unconscious world, to someone else's. Each one of us is truly unique in that way.

To give you an example; so far, the fastest I have ever had someone's water dramatically change is with my young son. His water changed size from a stream, to a lake, to an ocean, all within one 5 minute conversation. Again I didn't need to know why, I simply told him what to do with his water based on what he relayed to me that he was seeing in his mind moment to moment.

Many people have described some truly fascinating images in their water and organs when I work with them. Just be Ok with anything that shows up in your mind. It's all part of the process of unwinding things that are ready to be let go, for your emotional and/or physical benefit.

Now it's time to dive deeper into the water:

Again, ask your mind to show you an image of your water. Now, I want you to say to it;

I let go of everything and anything that is not mine.... I release it and set it free... and send it back to where it belongs, in peace. Thank You!

That's it. What happens? Does anything at all change in the image of your water?

Whatever happens or doesn't is fine.

Now say to your water;

I clear and remove any and all unwanted energy of any kind, known or unknown to me. I clear and remove any and all unwanted matter. And I fill in that space with peace.

What happens now, if anything at all? What are you aware of? What do you feel?

Now I want you to say to your water;

I bring sunbeams into every cell and every molecule of my entire body, to serve my greatest health and greatest good, in alignment for my optimal health.

What happens now? Just be the observer…What do you notice and feel? What is different.

Now say to your water;

For this moment now, I totally accept the love and the deep inner peace that aligns me and all the parts of me for my greatest health and greatest good… and I release anything and everything that is not that love or peace…for this moment now, I am at peace.

Take a deep breath in and out, and you are done for now.

Actually stop reading for 45 seconds and test out what you just read for yourself.

What changes, if anything? What are you aware of in your body? How do you feel?

When I work with clients, this dynamic process can get very involved, particularly as things change and unfold dynamically.

Allow yourself to be silent after you make a comment to your water. Allow whatever thought that might be deeper, to surface, and it will guide you as to what to do next.

My focus is to quiet my thinking mind, and to tap into a greater version of me in the silence. It is there that I know just what to do next, and so too can you. I am simply more practiced at this than you. Be patient with yourself and stay with this.

If you are at a loss as to what to do, just thank your water for what you want in advance.

Here are some simple examples of things that you might say to your water. Test out any or all of them and see what happens. Simply be the curious observer:

I love you and thank you for being there for me. I honor you commitment and I honor you. Thank You for helping me to heal fully.

Thank you for bringing moments of peace into my water, I love you.

Thank you for bringing light, playful moments into my water, I love you.

Thank you for bringing moments of joy throughin and throughout me. I love you.

Thank you for carrying the perfect healing molecules directly into the space that needs it. I love you and thank you so much.

Thank you for releasing and letting go exactly what is ready to be let go in perfect alignment for my greatest health and greatest good.

Thank you for eradicating, and clearing away, and removing anything that does not serve my greatest health and greatest good. I love you.

No time like the present moment to give a few of these a try. These are just ideas. Determine for yourself which ones have the most effect. Notice what works and what might have little to no perceivable effect. Tune into your feelings and inner intuition.

The specific ideas that I use with myself and clients comes from a place of knowing exactly what is needed. My outcome is always optimal health and inner balance and harmony. I am not sitting and concentrating or calculating what to do next. For me, the seamlessness flow of guidance comes from a deeper place. Allow that to develop from the silence that exists within you.

Be patient, kind, loving, tender and compassionate with yourself.

Under the Microscope

Unfortunately and fortunately, I was bitten in the leg by a highly toxic tick in late August of 2016. At the time I had no interest in writing a book on healing, as friends and family members were suggesting. I didn't want to revisit that long difficult health struggle by thinking about any of it.

But this little tick left a rather intense impression. Not only did I get the red bulls-eye rash that is characteristic of Lyme, I also got an infection and have the corresponding scar. I was beyond angry, as all I could think of was my previous years fighting with the disease.

By the way, to the best of my knowledge I was never bitten by a tick those many years ago when I struggled for so long. How then did I get Lyme? How is it that so many people who were never bitten by a tick have Lyme disease? The latest research suggests many other possibilities, and that may be a topic for another book.

Back to the tick bite, fortunately I knew exactly what to do.

Of course I went to my doctor to get Doxycycline, which is typically what the medical experts suggest, and what they usually give people who have the bulls-eye rash of Lyme. Often if Lyme is caught right away, a course of antibiotics will take care of the problem. In my case the antibiotics did absolutely nothing for me. I continued a downhill spiral and felt worse and worse until I gave up on the antibiotics and did my own thing.

Fortunately, I knew just what to do given my previous first-hand experience and understanding of the illness. But that can wait a bit because something fascinating happened.

What was fascinating to me was that when I looked at my water on the day after the tick bite, it was a dark black-red in color. It had never been that color ever in the previous year of looking at it.

I realized that I had lots of work to do to in order to restore the water to what had been a calm and completely crystal clear state. It had taken me a long time to get my water to that level of health.

This discovery was the catalyst for me to write this book.

I realized in that moment that people needed to know what to do, not just for Lyme, but for any chronic illness including cancer. I had been working with people with cancer for accelerating their healing, using the same ideas I used for my own Lyme, and with decent success.

Restoring balance and harmony in the body through the implementation of the ideas that you are reading about, seems to be potentially beneficial for most any illness.

My first line of healing repair for this toxic tick was an assortment of about a dozen anti-mircobials. I used them to deal with the infections and co-infections. Why I chose one over the other, and how I knew which ones to use and in what quantities was covered in Chapter 7.

I also worked diligently on my water and detox organs to speed my healing and clear die off from the bugs.

I began to feel better.

About four weeks in and feeling significantly improved, I had a thought about my water. It had been slowly clearing up with my work and was now a beige color.

I became curious about what I might see if I put the water under a microscope. As I super- magnified the image of water in my mind, getting deeper and deeper into the microscopic aspects of the water, I began to see three distinctly different types of bugs.

They were definitely something that needed to be addressed. What was I going to do about them?

As I sat in the silence connecting to my water; a sound tone appeared in my mind, and I had the idea that I could duplicate the sound tone and clean out the bugs.

I made the same tone out loud and watched as one of the types of bugs disintegrated, but the other bugs remained. Again, while waiting in the silence, a second and different tone surfaced.

I sounded that tone out loud, and all of the remaining bugs of one type were torn to pieces. I waited, and sure enough, a third distinctly different tone appeared in my mind. It was a little more difficult to duplicate the sound, but I was able to do it with a little effort.

The third variety of bug was obliterated. And there were no longer any bugs in my water. A few days later, I was able to get my water very close to back to the clarity that it had before the tick bite and I was feeling pretty normal.

Because I know what it's like to suffer for so many long years, I want people to have more useful tools to help themselves. These ideas absolutely helped me. If there is even a remote chance that you will benefit, put them into action right now, today. Do not let another day go by without testing them out for yourself. Any of these concepts and strategies can be implemented along with your current health protocols. They will not interfere with anything that you are already doing medically.

The Benefits of Sound

One of the things that I haven't mentioned so far is that I am a student of quantum physics. Not an official student of any sort, but someone who has attended seminars and read extensively on the subject. I like to keep up on the latest discoveries in quantum physics and similar areas. It's just an interest of mine, kind of like a hobby.

Some of what I do is consistent and connected to the science of quantum physics. There is so much to say about that, but I'm going to stick with sound for now.

Sound is simply a specific frequency. And different notes and tones of sound have different frequencies. That's why when you listen to different pieces of music, it will create different feelings for you. Sounds do influence us. The vast combinations of sound frequencies have varying impacts.

Scientists have been exploring the applications of sound for many years. Including applications where different sound frequencies can boil water, lift objects, and be used as military weapons. Interestingly, Middle Tennessee University recently discovered that some aspects of sound can travel faster than the speed of light.

By the way, scientists at the Department of Energy's Oak Ridge National Laboratory recently made a new discovery about water. It seems under certain conditions water molecules "tunnel". Basically, this means the molecules spread out when they are trapped in confined spaces, taking a new shape entirely. It's called quantum tunneling; a highly unexpected phenomenon.

There really is a great deal that we don't know or understand compared to what we do.

You may be aware that everything has a unique vibrational frequency, whether that's a person, a rock, a car, a pen, a maple leaf or a trout. We all have our own unique signature of vibrational signal.

Imagine a huge radio dial that gives you an infinite number of stations. When you move along the radio dial changing stations, you are also changing frequencies of vibration that correspond with specific things.

Ok, here's the point:

There are many electronic frequency devices available that can be useful in healing. In my opinion only, they don't always create healing, and they don't *always* create healing for *everyone*. My personal experience was a very limited benefit from using frequency devices.

Having said that, electronic frequency devices like Rife machines can be used to target specific types of organisms; like cancer cells, or specific Lyme spirochetes, or anything else. The device creates an offsetting frequency to whatever is targeted.

Basically that thing targeted with the frequency device is supposed to be killed by the offsetting frequency directed at it. Sometimes it happens, sometimes it doesn't.

The sound I created with my own voice tone was doing exactly that; it was targeting a specific type of Lyme bug, that had a specific type of frequency vibration, and the sound I made was able to obliterate it. Remember, I had to make three distinctly different sound tones to offset the three different types of bugs that I saw.

I have experimented with making sounds on cancer and other things.

Back to the skeptical part of you for a moment:

Where did the 3 different sounds that I heard in my mind come from? I believe that it's from divine inspiration, bubbling up from the silence of my mini-meditation while I connect with my water. Maybe it was my unconscious mind, or simply a much greater aspect of myself.

Did I just make the whole thing up in my mind? Remember back to the part about the unconscious mind? I simply trust what appears as real; obviously, with some degree of discernment. I have been working in clients unconscious worlds to resolve challenges for well over 10 years. I have a very good sense of how things work and function in that world.

Maybe the whole thing is just nonsense and not believable. That would mean that I am creating a healing placebo effect for myself, and the people that I have worked with. I would be happy with that actually happening. People feel better. I healed myself. What's the problem?

Would you say to the person who took the placebo sugar pill to cure their migraine; that even though they don't have the migraines anymore, and are healed, that the sugar pill didn't really work, and their migraines really aren't gone?

Speaking of placebos:

Numerous fake knee surgeries have been performed by a variety of orthopedic surgeons. The New England Journal of Medicine and the Wall St. Journal have both reported on placebo knee surgeries. What is really amazing is that very little difference in benefit exists in the outcomes of the fake vs. real knee surgery. This is wild to me.

What they do is sedate the patient, make an incision, do absolutely nothing inside the knee, they fix nothing, just sew the incision back up, and the patient believes that they had the full surgery. They don't' tell the patient it was fake until years later, following up on how they are doing.

The fake knee surgery people experience a similar decrease in discomfort, and increase in mobility and utilization etc...Amazingly, the two outcomes are similar in success. You can check this out for yourself online. It's more undeniable evidence of the placebo effect.

Your mind has incredible untapped power. We are the thing standing in the way of our own progress. We are the creator of our own limitations. We are the ones who doubt what we don't know and understand.

So, *Know* that you can heal! *Know* that amazing things are possible that you don't have to understand in order for them to actually work.

Know that you can facilitate and accelerate your own healing. *Know* that it can happen for you. And be willing to explore the possibilities of your own inner power by doing the things you are reading about.

Whether bringing love or peace into your water is what's working, or whether it's the placebo effect that is working for you, is completely irrelevant if you are in fact healing.

Choose to accept that there are many factors involved in true healing. There are causes of illness that the medical profession does fully not understand, so how could they possibly understand how to heal everyone, every time?

Frequently symptoms are treated instead of an active exploration to eliminate the source cause of the illness.

I believe that the work that you are reading about can help you to get at source causes. While it is also not perfect, it has proven to be highly beneficial for myself and many others.

Open your mind and give yourself and what you are reading an honest chance to work for you.

Find out for yourself by actual doing what you are reading with the corresponding level of effort that you deserve.

11

THE DYNAMICS PROCESS EXPANDS

To truly open your eyes and see for the very first time,
What is it that is real?

Expansion - Organs and Systems

There is a number of people that believe that organs and parts of the body have their own consciousness. Is this true? I have no idea. However, I do know that organs seem to respond to my work in a similar way as water.

I want you to imagine that you are able to shrink yourself down to a tiny level and go into your body and look at your heart. What do you see?

This simply requires a little imagination and your mind will do the rest.

Look around from this miniaturized you or simply imagine that you can see into your body and look at your heart. How does it look to you?

I began to do this to all of my organs and organ systems. My mind would give me an image that allowed me to interact with that particular organ. I believe this has been beneficial to accelerating the healing of that organ, using a similar approach as with the water.

Holographic Imaging

Here's an example:

I imagine looking at my heart in my mind's eye, and I am able to see an image that represents my heart. Is it real? What is real is that it seems to be a representation, like a holographic image, that simply represents my heart.

In this mind created, heart image, let's imagine that I see a shadow on the side of my heart, and I realize it doesn't belong. Do I need to do anything about it? Yes, because I want to have what looks like an optimal functioning of my heart, and a shadow isn't part of optimal functioning.

Is it an emotional shadow, or a physical, actual problem?

That doesn't matter to me. I simply want to know if I am able to remove the shadow. If so, my heart image will change and a beneficial shift will occur in my actual body. It might be subtle, it might be more significant, and it might take time for that to exist in my physical body.

Here's what you might do:

First make sure that you are in a silent undisturbed place. You want to slow down your thoughts and tune into your body.

Ask your mind to show you an image of your heart. Welcome the image of your heart. If you can't see anything, again, not a problem, simply do the exercise based on what FEELS right intuitively for you.

This could be the dialogue you direct to your heart (or any organ):

Be certain to talk to your heart or whatever organ you are interacting with, in an absolutely genuine tone. Have an attitude of gratitude that you are able to do this.

Relax, be at peace, slow down, take your time and feel the connectedness.

I want to thank you for being there for me,… for working so hard,… 24 hours a day,… sometimes I forget and I am so sorry…. Please forgive me…. I want you to know that I love you… and care about you… and appreciate you so much…Thank You!

In the silence simply observe the image of your heart, and notice if anything changes. If it does change great, if it doesn't, no worries.

Is that shadow still there? If you can't see your heart, do you sense that the shadow might still be there?

Tune into the silence and become aware of your own innate wisdom. Simply wait and observe your heart. There will be times when a thought will bubble up, and at other times, nothing.

Let's imagine that you sense or see nothing changing.

Now lets' say to your heart (or any other organ):

I release and let go of any and all unwanted energy…. I release and let go of everything and anything that is not mine…. I send it back to where it belongs, in peace… Thank You!

I have done this to my body, and every organ and system that I can think of. I have found it helpful to remove shadows or residue, and things of that sort.

To continue: (remember, simply be the curious observer)

I allow love and peace to flow freely… throughin and throughout me…clearing away blocks to my healing…removing anything that doesn't serve my greatest health…allowing the re-ordering of molecules into perfect balance and harmony… for my greatest good… Thank You!

What happened? Did anything shift or change or respond in any way in the image of your heart or (whatever organ you directed this to)? Did you notice any feeling change in your body?

To continue further:

"I sweep clear any trauma… or transgression from the past… allowing the optimal level of energy to flow…restoring full balance and harmony…for my greatest health…and greatest good…I release any and all unnecessary protectiveness that might exist from a misunderstanding or trauma…and I honor my ability and willingness to re-align in perfect order and function for my greatest health.

Now it's time to evaluate. What changed in the image? How do you feel? Are you aware of any emotional changes in you? Do you feel lighter?

When I work with myself or clients, this process evolves naturally based on the dynamic, holographic image changes that are seen in the mind. Trust in the process. Trust your unconscious imaging. Trust your intuition and inner knowingness.

Be Ok with whatever emotions might come up.

It's perfectly normal if you feel like crying for a few moments. Sometimes emotional releases occur. They typically only last a few moments as things are let go.

Be sincere. Be genuine. Allow yourself to reflect truthfully on how this feels for you. Honor the unknown aspects of yourself that can enhance your healing. Be at peace in these small moments of self-nurturing.

Work with your body, organs, and water once a day or a few times a day, nothing more than that. I personally never did this more than 2x in a day, and mostly just 1x/day, but I did it for 5-15 minutes depending

on what seemed to feel right. As time goes on, you will have a deeper sense of what is needed. Trust in your own innate wisdom, and allow yourself to be guided, perhaps for some, even divinely guided as to what more you need to do for yourself.

12

SPACE AND FIELDS

*Advanced technologies are giving us
a glimpse into the previous unknown.*

There is so much more to be understood.

The science of quantum physics and quantum mechanics is changing our perspective about everything. Albert Einstein said, *"We still do not know one thousandth of one percent of what nature has revealed to us."*

Recently the National Academy of Science revealed that 99.9% of all life forms on the earth have yet to be discovered. Biologists believe that they have discovered less than 25% of all plants and animals on the earth, and 95% of the ocean remains unexplored.

So much of what surrounds us is unknown to us. While those are examples of our physical world, the invisible world that surrounds us is even more complex and unknown.

Life Energy

For thousands of years ancient cultures have believed that an energetic flow exists within the body. The ancient Chinese called it Chi, the Japanese called it Ki, the Hindu's called it Prana, and the ancient Greeks called it Pneuma.

These cultures and many Indigenous tribes all over the world have believed for thousands of years, that this vital life energy circulated in and around the body, and could be utilized in healing.

The Energy Field of the Heart

- Research by the Institute for HeartMath in California has shown that the heart's electrical field is about 60 times greater than the electrical activity of the brain.
- The magnetic field produced by the heart is over 5000 times stronger than the field generated by the brain.
- The electromagnetic energy of the heart not only envelops every cell of the human body, but also extends out in all directions into the space around us.
- Our heart field touches those within 8 - 10 feet of where we are positioned (and perhaps in more subtle ways at greater distances).

In my opinion, this profound information is the beginning of understanding the role that the heart and emotions can play in accelerating healing.

Space

Super-powered electron microscopes are now allowing scientists to discover particle sizes that were not known to exist just 5 years ago. Our understanding of ourselves, the earth, and the Universe continues to evolve.

Scientists can measure the human electrical and bio-energy fields, as well as the electromagnetic fields of the brain and heart. NASA and a number of research scientists have identified something known as *Quantum Foam*, which is the teeniest, tiniest, sea of the minutest particles yet discovered. These particles blink in and out of existence at astonishing speeds.

Ok, what's this have to do with health? Stay with me, this science background is relevant to my healing process.

It seems that there is no such thing as empty space, there is only something like *quantum foam* everywhere at the deepest level of the space. And at the most minute level, the human body is mostly *quantum foam*.

If we take something as small as the nucleus of an atom, and magnify it up to the size of a marble, the outer ring of the atom would appear the size of a football stadium surrounding that marble. Everything else inside the ring of the stadium is space, previously thought to be empty now known to contain this *quantum foam* like substance.

We are a microcosm of the Universe. Imagine the distances between stars and galaxies. Similar ratios of distance exist between the minutest particles within us. The rest is space, filled with something that resembles *quantum foam*.

Here are a few important considerations to know that relate to this Healing System:

- The Human body is surrounded by an energy field.
- The heart's electromagnetic field is 60x greater than the brain's.
- Can these energy fields be utilized in healing?
- At the most extreme levels of magnification we are 99% space, but that space might have an intelligence and aliveness of its' own.
- Can that space be utilized in healing?

Balancing the Fields

I believe that when energy fields and systems become unbalanced, that illness can occur. This is simply my personal opinion. Some of my own healing work was directed at rebalancing and harmonizing my body's subtle energy fields.

This process is similar to talking with your water and organs. Which we will do right now;

Ready?

Take a look at your water in your mind's eye before doing this process. Notice how your water appears to you. Notice the color, shape, size, clarity, and surroundings if any…

Now we are going to talk to our energy field, and do a little experiment to see if talking to our energy field has any impact on our water.

Simple enough right?

Imagine that you are surrounded by a field of flowing energy, direct this thought out loud or silently into your energy field. Take 7 or 8 seconds and do this slowly and genuinely. Now say:

I love you… and thank you for being there for me… I appreciate all you do for me… Thank You.

Remember to FEEL grateful.

Ok, now take a look at your water. Did anything change or shift it its' appearance? Do you feel any different in any subtle way?

Of course you actually did this, right?

This process can easily expand just as it does with your water and organs:

Now say any or all of the following to your energy field:

- *I release any and all tangles in my energy field…restoring perfect divine order.*
- *I balance and harmonize my energy fields… for my greatest health and greatest good.*
- *I repair any and all imbalances,… tears… and imperfections in my energy fields…restoring perfect balance and harmony.*
- *I bring love into my energy field…. I bring peace into my energy field.*
- *I stop all fluxing and fluttering in my field …and restore perfect operating order… in divine alignment… for my greatest health and greatest good.*

Now quickly take another look at the image of your water in your mind. Did anything change? Is anything different? And do you feel different at all in any subtle way?

I am always curious about what I am able to observe that is different before and after doing any of these processes. When things or feelings change and shift, even in the most subtle of ways, I know that I am on the right track. And so are you.

You could add working with your energy field for as little as 30 seconds after working with your water. Tap into your own intuition to sense what your body might need focus on. Honor your own sense of knowing and trust your instincts and inner wisdom.

The more you honor and trust that part of you that knows what is needed, the stronger it will become. All it takes is a willingness to listen in the silence after asking what your body, organ, water, or field might need, and wait to see what surfaces in your mind.

Energy Centers

Ancient wisdom also believes that the body has Energy Centers or wheels of life located both inside and outside the body. The Chinese identified these various centers as *dantien*. The best known is the Hindu system, and the word *chakra* from Sanskrit which means wheel. There are thought to be 7 primary chakras.

Imagine them as wheels of energy. Here are the basic locations:

1. Root Chakra — Location: Base of spine in tailbone area.

2. Sacral Chakra — Location: Lower abdomen, about two inches below the navel

3. Solar Plexus Chakra — Location: Upper abdomen in the stomach area.

4. Heart Chakra — Location: Center of chest just above the heart.

5. Throat Chakra — Location: Throat

6. Third Eye Chakra — Location: Forehead between the eyes.

7. Crown Chakra — Location: The very top of the head.

In my mind I imagine looking at the energy centers and simply notice what appears. In the past, I have seen gray streaks in an energy center, a variety of imbalances, muddled appearances, or something I can't identify that seems out of order.

Then, I simply do similar types of things as with my water, or organs or field.

For example you might say to your energy centers:

I love you.

I bring perfect balance and harmony into all of my energy centers.

I clear away any and all unwanted energy in my energy centers.

I bring divine love and light into this energy center to lighten and brighten in perfect balance and harmony… for my greatest health and greatest good.

Typically, I include working on my energy centers along with the work on my field, based solely on my intuition about what might be needed.

For example:

- *I bring peace into my field and energy centers.*
- *I bring love into my field and energy centers.*
- *I bring perfect balance and harmony into my fields and energy centers.*
- *I clear and remove any and all unwanted energy from my fields and energy centers.*
- *I release and let go of any shadows and traces of trauma from my field and energy centers.*
- *I align my fields and energy centers in perfect divine order for my greatest health and greatest good.*

Utilizing the Space

I consider space to be a creative and intelligent aspect of the divine that can be utilized for healing. That's simply my opinion.

These opinions that you've been reading about form the foundation of the tools and strategies that I use to accelerate healing. Since you are now aware of how I work with water, and a little about the fields and energy centers, the space is simply a deeper layer.

To keep things simple: Imagine that you are simply looking through a super microscope and going deeper and deeper into the layers of water where nothing exists except space.

Here's what I do that you can do for yourself:

Just as directing specific thoughts or dialogue into the water, field and energy centers, you will now direct the thoughts into the space that you are. You can do this out loud or quietly in your mind. There is no difference.

Example:

"Into this water I bring love", can evolve to *"Into this space that I am, I bring love."*

Now stop for a moment and try it out for yourself. Imagine saying deep into the heart of your space. *"Into this space that I am, I bring love. "*

See what happens; notice what you feel… if anything.

Say to your space any of the following things, but one at a time. Take your time, and be genuine with feeling and gratitude.

Intentionally focus on the deepest aspect of yourself, and notice whatever you notice, and feel whatever you feel without judgment, simply curiosity:

- *Into this space that I am, I bring love.*
- *Into this space that I am, I bring deep soothing peace.*
- *Into this space I bring love and light.*
- *I re-orient this space into perfect balance and harmony for my greatest health.*
- *I re-balance and re-order this space for my greatest health and greatest good.*

- *I clear and remove any and all unwanted energy and unwanted matter from my space …allowing only that which serves my greatest health and greatest good.*
- *Into this space, I bring the creative love and light of the divine… nurturing this space and returning to perfect divine order.*
- *I release and let go any unwanted clustering and tangles that do not serve my greatest health.*
- *I lighten and brighten my space into perfect divine alignment.*

You can of course combine the field, energy centers, and space into one directive. Again, I access my own inner knowingness about what is needed in any particular connection with my body and energy systems. I trust my unconscious mind or divine guidance to bring me insights into what is needed.

For Example:

- *I release and let go any unwanted energy from my field, my energy centers and my space …restoring perfect balance and harmony for my greatest health and greatest good.*
- *I thank my field, my energy centers and my space for aligning in perfect healing balance and harmony… for my greatest good.*
- *I stop any and all fluttering in my field…, my energy centers… and my space… restoring perfect balance and harmony… for my greatest health and greatest good.*
- *I release and let go of any and all anger and rage… (Fill in your favorite disempowering emotions) from my field, my energy centers and my space. (shame, humiliation, despair, pain, hopelessness, guilt, grief, sadness, injustice, terror, fear, bitterness, resentment, etc…*

By the way, injustice is definitely an emotion to release and let go. It holds a strong energetic charge that you want eliminate.

Our water, organs, DNA, systems, fields, energy centers and space hold things that do not serve us. It can be helpful to let go of any negative emotions that you can think of.

If you were to think about all of the negative emotional experiences that you've had in your life, there are probably plenty to be let go. Tune into whatever area of your body and or field etc…that you are working on, and sense if a particular emotion is ready to be let go.

Always thank whatever area you are working on and know that every aspect of you wants to return to complete balance, harmony and optimal health. Every part of you is on your side.

Things occasionally get out of alignment because of any host of things including emotional traumas, physical ailments, collective consciousness, environmental issues, human dynamics, spiritual misalignment, lack of purpose, etc…

We are all just a work in progress doing the best we can in any moment of time.

13

50 RULES FOR HEALTHY LIVING

Live fully, Love completely,
and Pursue the things that really matter.

Examine your life within the context of these *50 Rules for Healthy Living*. Perhaps you will find an area or two that needs something more from you.

1. An aliveness and enthusiasm for life.
2. A sense of curiosity and adventure
3. A willingness to forgo short-term gratification in support of a bigger plan.
4. A capacity to genuinely love and be loved.
5. A willingness to be friends with and interact harmoniously with people.
6. A sense of purpose in living.
7. A determined attitude of positivity.
8. A welcoming of personal growth and change.
9. A willingness to give to others freely.
10. A natural state of living.
11. A community and communion of connections to share the variables of life.
12. A sense of wonder and awe about life.

13. A void of negativity and negative interactions.
14. A willingness to truly embrace peaceful moments.
15. A moderation of food and exercise.
16. A connection to the Divine.
17. A focus away from self.
18. A giving, growing, learning, sharing cycle of life embraced.
19. An ability to let go of transgressions committed to and by.
20. A nurturing approach to self.
21. A dominant understanding of serving something greater than self.
22. An attitude of gratitude and thankfulness.
23. A sense of humor and lightness about life.
24. A sense of optimism about the future
25. An ability to overcome and find peace in tragedy and adversity.
26. A welcoming heart.
27. An internal system of honor and integrity
28. Divine guidance welcomed.
29. Gestures of kinship without judgment.
30. Fortitude and an insightful approach to path of choice.
31. Creativity expressed.
32. Novelty embraced.
33. A breakaway understanding of societal norms that distract primary focus.
34. A methodical approach to living, with habits and rituals that support life.
35. Troubles forgotten.
36. Inspiration breathed daily.
37. A timeless mind and playfulness integrated into life.
38. Constructs of Divinity surrounding
39. An approach to health and healing with ease and grace.
40. Practical applied daily action.
41. An avoidance of danger in all forms.

42. Traditions honored and treasured, or created.
43. A living attitude of possibility.
44. A relaxed focus.
45. A moderation of emotional living.
46. A primary desire to share love in some form.
47. Timeless wisdom adopted.
48. Pursuits fully embraced.
49. An adventurous and generous spirit.
50. An opportunistic heart willing to give and share.

There is truly timeless wisdom in these *50 Rules for Healthy Living*. What specifically are you willing to do differently in your life? When will that start?

What promise will you make to yourself right here, and right now?

What from this list of *50 Rules* will be added to your own healing plan?

14

SUMMARY

*An awakening beyond our current understanding
is sometimes necessary in order to heal fully and completely.*

An awakening beyond my understanding was necessary for me. Many aspects of my life needed to be upgraded. My existing programming had run out of its' usefulness. I found my path and my purpose through my healing journey. You can do the same thing.

Our greatest wisdom comes from our greatest struggles in life. We cannot grow without adversity. This I know only too well.

In the times we are most tested are the times we grow the most. Allow the wisdom from your very personal healing journey, to blaze a happier and more fulfilling path for you. Reach out for support when you need it.

Be patient with yourself. Treat yourself with kindness and compassion. We are all quite good at beating ourselves up. Allow yourself to receive love, particularly your own, and work to elevate your level of Self-Love and Self-Acceptance.

Here are some reminders:

✓ Upgrade your thoughts and feelings to something elevating to your mood and life experience.

✓ Upgrade your nutritional intake to a level that elevates your body's ability to heal.

✓ Upgrade your physical movement to be more active with your body.

✓ Upgrade your environmental awareness. Pay attention to what's around you in all aspects of life; including social media, TV and mindless unhealthy distractions.

✓ Upgrade your Life Balance, and cut out the activities, distractions, and unhealthy immersions that do not serve you long term.

✓ Upgrade your Interactions with all the people in your life. There may be some people that need to be let go.

✓ Upgrade your understanding about what will be most beneficial to your future health maintenance.

✓ Continue to practice accessing what FEELS right for you. Use moments of silence or brief quiet contemplation, to enhance your intuition and wisdom.

✓ Slow your life down by being more deeply involved in whatever you are doing. Do not multi-task. It's ineffective, and keeps you locked into your thinking mind. That won't serve you long term. Your intuitive feeling heart and instinctive gut, will provide better guidance.

✓ Take an honest look at your life. Do you know your purpose? Does your life have meaning in a way that fulfills you? What compelling things are you looking forward to?

There is so much more to say from the work that I do with the Magenta Healing Systems including additional systems that are much more complex. What you have read here is more than enough to help you to

accelerate your own healing as it was for me. It is also only the beginning. These other systems and discoveries will be covered in another book, or in another way. I continue to receive evolutionary, divine healing wisdom from within the silence of my mini-mediations. I will be sharing all of that in due time.

The next level:

An awakening beyond your current understanding.

Catalyst Rising- *The Art of Self and Group Healing, Through the Magenta Healing Systems.*

You can reach me at jeff@peakresultscoaching.com or visit www.peakresultscoaching.com Schedule a conversation to talk with me if you are ready to explore having my support in your healing journey. I look forward to hearing from you.

Wishing you all the best in health!

Jeff Forte

PEAK Results Coaching

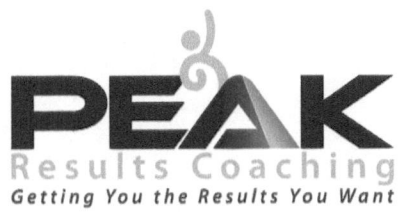

www.ingramcontent.com/pod-product-compliance
Lightning Source LLC
Chambersburg PA
CBHW020537290526
45786CB00002B/930